OPERATIVE TECHNIQUES IN PLASTIC SURGERY
Series Editor
John M. Goin, M.D.
Emeritus Clinical Professor of Surgery (Plastic)
USC School of Medicine
Los Angeles, California

Color Atlas of SMAS Rhytidectomy

Mark L. Lemmon, M.D.
Clinical Assistant Professor
Division of Plastic Surgery
University of Texas
Southwestern Medical Center
Dallas, Texas

1993
Thieme Medical Publishers, Inc. NEW YORK
Georg Thieme Verlag STUTTGART • NEW YORK

Thieme Medical Publishers, Inc.
381 Park Avenue South
New York, New York 10016

Library of Congress Cataloging-in-Publication Data

Lemmon, Mark L. (Mark Leonard), 1924–
Color atlas of SMAS rhytidectomy / Mark L. Lemmon.
p. cm. — (Operative techniques in plastic surgery)
Includes bibliographical references and index.
ISBN 0-86577-485-4 (Thieme Medical Publishers). — ISBN (invalid)
3-13-109801-1 (G. Thieme Verlag)
1. Facelift—Atlases. I. Title. II. Series.
[DNLM: 1. Rhytidoplasty—methods—atlases. WE 17 L554c 1993]
RD119.5.F33L45 1993
617.5′20592—dc20
DNLM/DLC
for Library of Congress 93-8232
CIP

Important note: Medicine is an ever-changing science. Research and clinical experience are continually broadening our knowledge, in particular our knowledge of proper treatment and drug therapy. Insofar as this book mentions any dosage or application, readers may rest assured that the authors, editors, and publishers have made every effort to ensure that such references are strictly in accordance with the state of knowledge at the time of production of the book. Nevertheless, every user is requested to carefully examine the manufacturers' leaflets accompanying each drug to check on his own responsibility whether the dosage schedules recommended therein or the contraindications stated by the manufacturers differ from the statements made in the present book. Such examination is particularly important with drugs that are either rarely used or have been newly released on the market.

Printed in the United States of America.

5 4 3 2 1

TMP ISBN 0-86577-485-4
GTV ISBN 3-13-109801-1

ACKNOWLEDGMENTS

I am grateful to William M. Winn, Director, Medical Creative Services, Scottish Rite Children's Center, Atlanta, Georgia, for his talented production of the line drawings interpreting and illustrating the techniques and photographs of this book.

Also a dedicated contributor is Michael Lorfing, President of Synapse, Inc., who throughout the photographing of the operative procedures always strove to obtain the highest quality of photograph, and uniformity of framing to satisfy the intent of this book.

Over the years many have served in various capacities in the production and typing of the manuscripts—thanks particularly to Mary Chapman and Dianne Powell.

Thanks to Patricia Melton. She prepared the way in the operating room, making each day simpler and more pleasant—and more efficient.

Rebecca Rogers, who prepared the manuscript, and patiently and promptly responded to each request, deserves my appreciation and thanks.

CONTENTS

FOREWORD

Tord Skoog, for many years Professor of Plastic Surgery at the University of Uppsala, has undeservedly faded from the para-Jungian collective consciousness of the present generation of American plastic surgeons. The plastic surgical pantheon has a replacement rate roughly equal to that of a Marine infantry platoon on Iwo Jima in February, 1945.

This unpretentious, self-effacing, highly-gifted, Swedish surgeon was one of the titans during my own formative years as a plastic surgeon. I learned more from him while sitting in hotel bars at conventions than I did from many a teaching course or scientific session. His surgical interests were protean: inverted nipples, rhinolalia, mammary hypertrophy, hypospadias, nasal deformities, clefts of the lip and alveolus, the aging face; there was an original, and usually ingenious, Skoog operation for all of these. His facelift, I would urge, was one of his most important and lasting contributions to facial plastic surgery.

Mark Lemmon fell under Skoog's spell, as did I and many other American plastic surgeons; two names that come to mind are Rex Peterson, one of the first and best products of what was to become the UCLA residency, and Jack Owsley, a co-resident from my UCSF days. They, and others too numerous to mention, expanded on Skoog's revolutionary operation (based on the SMAS, which would not be 'discovered' for many years), refined it, and fine-tuned it.

I have always felt a special attraction to Mark Lemmon's (and Sam Hamra's) logical and gradually-achieved modifications of this operation based always on sound anatomical principles, partly because they initially almost exactly paralleled, and eventually far exceeded, my own attempts to surpass the master. And partly, and more importantly, because Lemmon's technique is safe (given a clear understanding of the anatomy), effective, adaptable, and notably free from gimmickry.

At the risk of turning this appreciation of Mark Lemmon's work into an autobiography, let me digress briefly on my own training. Our residency was both blessed and cursed by its association with an entity I'll call the Samuel Plotkin Foundation, which provided residents with an almost unlimited number of aesthetic surgical patients, an unusual circimstance in those days. Mr. Plotkin was an extremely successful businessman whose interest in aesthetic surgery bordered on the obsessive. Through his charitable foundation he would interview 'deserving' Southern Californian women and, if they met certain criteria at which I can only guess, he would underwrite their hospital bills. These trusting souls would arrive at our clinic with detailed instructions from Mr. Plotkin: 'shorten nose 1/4",' 'erase smile lines but don't smooth forehead too much,' 'eliminate downturning lines at corners of mouth and plump out cheeks by 25%,' and so on. We residents thought these little prescriptions were a hoot. We did not discriminate among facelift patients since we knew what to do. Squirt the local anesthetic into the inadequately sedated patient's face. Cope with shrieks and tears by adopting the formula of the aristocratic foreign Fellow, 'Kindly compose yourself, madame.' Then the same methylene blue markings made without regard to variations in the hairline or anything else. Cut along the line, push and shove with the scissors, stop the bleeding, pull the skin as tight as possible with Kocher clamps, cut off the excess and sew 'em up. What a bore! Where were all the cleft lips and total nasal reconstructions? The real operations.

Samuel Plotkin's mad idea that a facelift could be tailored to deal with a specific patient's aging changes just went to show what happened when a furniture dealer, in his ignorance, tried to meddle in surgical matters.

Well, eventually most of us figured out that Mr. Plotkin was on the right track after all. A facelift needn't be the paint-by-the-numbers operation that was commonly done in those days; a negative vestige, perhaps, of our general surgical training. It was a 'real operation' after all. Mark Lemmon was among the first in this country to grasp these fundamental ideas: that the skin-only facelift was, with rare exceptions, a thing of the past; and that the procedure could and should be individualized according to the needs of the patient, just as we were learning to do with rhinoplasties.

That all surgery has its foundation in anatomy is a truism never too obvious to repeat. Mark Lemmon's precise anatomical studies, and the magnificent pictures that illustrate them, epitomize this cliché. Each and every aspect of his operation springs from his intimate knowledge of the architecture of the face and neck. Readers searching for a safe, anatomically sound facelift technique which provides reproducible results, is adaptable to any case, and will produce excellent and (provided the patient has been selected properly) long-lasting results need look no further. This book deserves careful, line-by-line, illustration-by-illustration study. There are no fillers. Only facts derived from a long, thoughtful, scientific, and self-critical experience.

John M. Goin, M.D.
Series Editor

PREFACE

Timothy Ferris, in excerpts from his book *The Mind's Sky: Human Intelligence in a Cosmic Context*, (*New York Times Magazine*, December 15, 1991), proposes that the role of harmony in biological evolution has been underestimated. Darwinism stresses fierceness and competition. Ferris suggests "to be fit" means not so much that "it (the individual) can dominate others but that it is attuned to its environment. . . . It just may be that human beings and other organisms are selected in part on what might be called esthetic grounds . . . because they felt they belonged here—were able to enjoy life, to resonate with the world."[1] The face is the visible epicenter of belonging, and the aging face is a loss of belonging.

Since Noel performed the first wedge excision of the scalp in an attempt to improve facial aesthetics, the search has continued unabated for a better operation to improve the appearance of aging of the face and neck. Because of this, facelift procedures extended more widely, and eventually the limits of subdermal dissection were reached and thought to be the ultimate result. For the few, depending on skin-type genetics, such procedures can produce excellent and long-term results. But for the many, the quality of results was shortlived. Thus accepted by most as the limit of face-lifting, the boundaries of a skin facelift were only lightly questioned until Skoog[2] in 1969 opened the door to a procedure based on surgical anatomy. Mitz and Peyronie's description[3] of the superficial musculoaponeurotic system (SMAS)-platysma muscle provided the anatomical basis for a restoration of the anatomy of the face.

It seems worthwhile to point out some significant initial events in the evolution of the SMAS-platysma facelift. In 1973 at Baker and Gordon's annual symposium on cosmetic surgery, Skoog[4] presented and demonstrated the sub-SMAS facelift, which in 1969 he had referred to as a "useful technique in face-lifting"[2] in a presentation at the annual meeting of the American Association of Plastic Surgeons in San Francisco. The procedure described was based on the anatomy of the head and neck and sound surgical principles—mobilization of the involved tissues, advancement, and repair. The objective was twofold—improvement of the nasolabial folds and elimination of the skin–platysma muscle folds of the neck. The dissection of the cheek extended to the nasolabial fold, but did not totally release all the tissues extending to the nasolabial fold. In addition, the dissection described, while presented as sub-SMAS, was not completely sub-SMAS, as anteriorly (medial) it was superficial to the zygomaticus muscles. Recently Barton[5] defined this very well. Suffice to say that in the cheek, except for the extent and the complete release of the tissues to the nasolabial fold and better definition of the anatomy of the area, today's procedures are little different than those described by Skoog.

The neck was another matter and early on it was clear that SMAS-platysma muscle advancement did not eliminate the skin–platysma muscle folds of the neck. Guerrero-Santos[6–9] and Connell[10,11] described direct approaches for correction of the platysma muscle folds of the neck. Millard and his coworkers[12–14] described lipectomies of the submental-cervical region, which combined with myectomy of the anterior borders of the platysma muscle added immensely to contouring of the neck.

I am indebted to John Goin, for providing the opportunity to present a technique for rhytidectomy, which, in his words, is "the way you do it." Without his encouragement, guidance, and patience, this work would not have come to fruition.

The procedure described in this work is an extensive elevation of the SMAS extending to and slightly medial to the nasolabial fold and a restoration of the cervicomental angle by platysma muscle and lipectomy in the region, if indicated. Experience has proven the procedure to be constantly reproducible and reliable when matched against the myriad of aging changes in the face and neck presented to the surgeon. Experience also has shown that less than the described procedure falls short of expected results. Mastery and confidence in this procedure should serve one well and prepare the way for whatever may or may not prove to be future generations of rhytidectomy.[15]

No attempt has been made to compare the procedure in this work with works of the many successful plastic surgeons who have contributed greatly to the evolution of the rhytidectomy that incorporates SMAS-platysma muscle restoration, and cervical lipectomies and adjunctive procedures of the lower face. Nor does the text discuss an array of complications and their management except at this point to state that they are equal, or less than the known acceptable limits, and in most areas the results of the sub-SMAS and cervical restoration far exceed results possible with lesser procedures that have an equal or greater number of complications.

Beside the basic technique of the management of the SMAS and the platysma muscle, there are many nuances of rhytidectomy related to the skin—incisions, redraping, and trimming of the excess tissue—and such things as organization of the sequence of the procedure, all of which add to the finished product. As the text moves with the atlas illustrations, it will take note of these small but important aspects of the procedure.

Without too much redundancy or oversimplification, the rhytidectomy technique is presented by text and by illustrations and photographs, including fresh cadaver dissection and intraoperative views, in parallel. Each of these has its limitations and its advantages, but together they complement each other and, hopefully, as a whole provide a better understanding. Where a single illustration or photograph sufficed to demonstrate a point, parallel presentation was not used. In some vital areas of the procedure, a parallel presentation was considered necessary although the point might seem obvious with less.

A final word—mastery of a stimulating exercise in anatomical dissection and repair can provide great satisfaction to the operator. Even when the procedure is beautifully performed, there are limitations. But when combined with dutiful, detailed preoperative preparation of the patient, it offers the best opportunity for long-term successful results and for a patient who understands the limitations of human tissues—specifically theirs.

Emotional preparation and anatomical repair of the face and neck restore the sense of belonging—the ability "to resonate with the world."[1]

Mark L. Lemmon, M.D.

References

1. Ferris, T.: A cosmological event. New York Times Magazine. New York Times Co. December 15, 1991, p. 53.
2. Skoog, T.: Useful techniques in face lifting. Presented at the meeting of the American Association of Plastic Surgeons, San Francisco, CA, April 1969.
3. Mitz, V. and Peyronie, M.: The superficial musculoaponeurotic system (SMAS) in the parotid and cheek area. Plast. Reconstr. Surg. 1976; 58:80–88.
4. Skoog, T.: Rhytidectomy: A personal experience and technique. Presented and demonstrated on live television at the Seventh Annual Symposium on Cosmetic Surgery at the Cedars of Lebanon Hospital, Miami, FL, February 1973.
5. Barton, F.E.: The SMAS and the nasolabial fold. Plast. Reconstr. Surg. 1992; 89:1054–1059.
6. Guerrero-Santos, J.: Muscular flap in cervical rhytidoplasty. Presented at the annual meeting of the American Society of Plastic and Reconstructive Surgeons, Hollywood, FL, October 1973.
7. Guerrero-Santos, J.: Face lift surgical technique. Presented at the annual symposium on Aesthetic-Plastic Surgery, Guadalajara, Mexico, October 1974.
8. Guerrero-Santos, J.: The role of the platysma muscle in rhytidectomy. Clin. Plast. Surg. 1978; 5:29–49.
9. Guerrero-Santos, J., Spaillat, L., and Morales, F.: Muscular lift in cervical rhytidectomy. Plast. Reconstr. Surg. 1974; 54:127–131.
10. Connell, B.F.: Cervical lifts: The value of platysma muscle flaps. Ann. Plast. Surg. 1978; 1:32–43.
11. Connell, B.F.: Contouring the neck in rhytidectomy by lipectomy and muscle sling. Plast. Reconstr. Surg. 1978; 61:376–383.
12. Millard, D.R.: Plastic peregrinations. Plast. Reconstr. Surg. 1950; 5:26–53.
13. Millard, D.R., et al.: Submental and submandibular lipectomy in conjunction with a face lift in the male or female. Plast. Reconstr. Surg. 1972; 49: 385–391.
14. Millard, D.R., Pigott, R.W., and Hedo, S.: Submandibular lipectomy. Plast. Reconstr. Surg. 1968; 41:513–522.
15. Hamra, S.T.: Composite rhytidectomy. Plast. Reconstr. Surg. 1992; 90: 1–13.

ONE

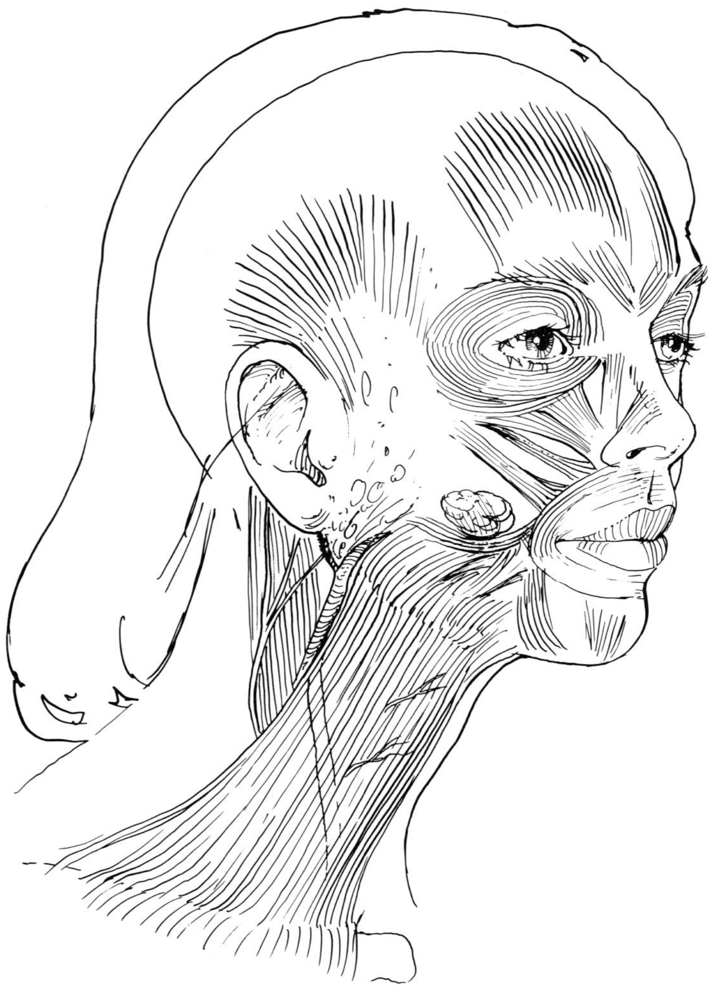

The Surgical Anatomy of the SMAS Rhytidectomy

The operator's confidence and success in a SMAS-platysma muscle rhytidectomy depends on a thorough knowledge and familiarity with the intricate anatomy of the head and neck. Of particular importance is the anatomy of the superficial and deep fasciae of the cheek. While constant, it varies immensely in morphologic development and quality, and the myriad of conditions encountered by the surgeon range from thin to fat faces, weak to strong tissues, and poorly or well-defined tissue planes. The reassurance of the surgeon, as well as the progress and efficiency of the procedure, is enhanced immensely upon mastery of the anatomy of region and the superficial and deep fasciae of the cheek.

The surgical anatomy of the aging face is a result of the more mobile, kinetic superficial fascia's loss of elasticity and its resultant attenuation. The variation in the degree of relaxation in various portions of the superficial musculoaponeurotic system (SMAS), combined with areas of greater fixation between the superficial and deep fasciae, causes deepening of the nasolabial folds, jowl formation, and platysma muscle folds of the face and neck. The result is a loss of the younger contours of the face and neck as well as diminution in the dynamics of facial expression.

Fig. 1–1 illustrates the structures that compose the SMAS. The cadaver dissections[1] (Figs. 1–2, 1–3, and 1–4) demonstrate the anatomical relationships of the muslces (orbicularis oculi, zygomaticus major and minor, and platysma muscles) that are contained in the superficial fascia. In vivo the zygomatic-nasolabial fold area (see Fig. 1–2) has a covering of fibrous fatty tissue. This has been removed to demonstrate the underlying musculature. In this area the skin and subcutaneous fat are elevated superficial to the zygomaticus major and minor muscles (superficial to the SMAS) whereas elsewhere in a SMAS rhytidectomy the superficial fascia is elevated.[2]

Fig. 1–3 demonstrates the superficial musculature of the face without the fascial or aponeurotic portion of the SMAS. The removal of the superficial and deep fasciae discloses the facial nerve branches anterior to the parotid gland, and particularly the buccal branches crossing the buccal fat pad,

Figure 1–1. Structural components of the SMAS.

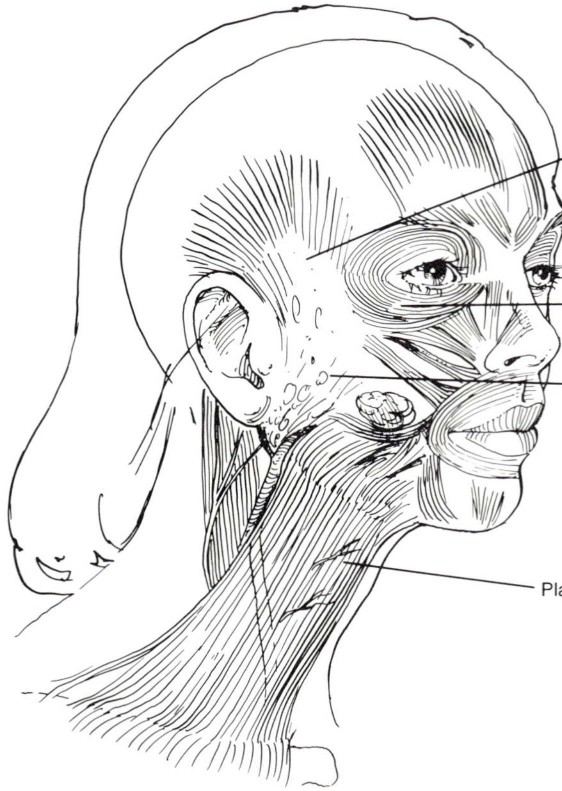

Figure 1–2. SMAS rhytidectomy: The orbital zygomatic musculature. 12 = frontal belly of occipitofrontalis; 13 = orbital part of orbicularis oculi; 14 = palpebral part of orbicularis oculi; 15 = medial palebral ligament; 16 = depressor supercilii; 17 = procerus; 18 = nasalis; 19 = angular vein; 20 = levator labii superioris alaeque nasi; 21 = levator labii superioris; 22 = levator anguli oris; 23 = facial artery; 24 = facial vein; 25 = zygomaticus minor; 26 = zygomaticus major; 27 = buccal branches of facial nerve; 28 = zygomatic branches of facial nerve.

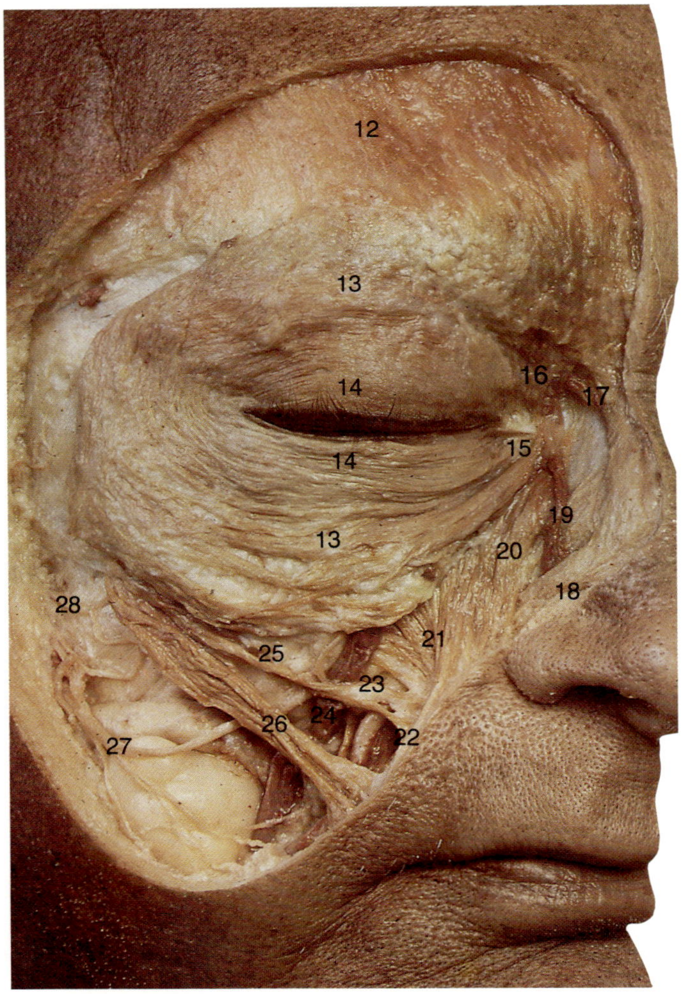

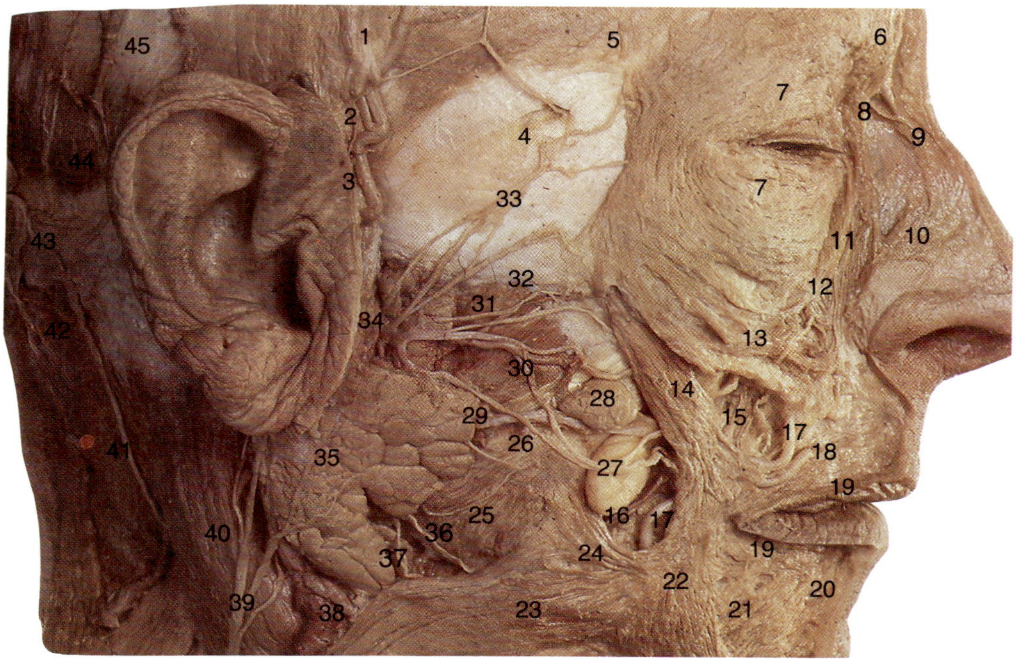

Figure 1–3. SMAS rhytidectomy: The anatomy of the cheek (The right parotid gland, facial nerve, and facial muscles [with removal of the upper part of the parotid gland]). 1 = temporoparietalis; 2 = auriculotemporal nerve; 3 = superficial temporal artery; 4 = zygomaticotemporal nerve piercing temporalis fascia; 5 = epicranial aponeurosis (galea aponeurotica); 6 = frontal belly of occipitofrontalis; 7 = orbicularis oculi; 8 = depressor supercilii; 9 = procerus; 10 = nasalis; 11 = levator labii superioris alaeque nasi; 12 = levator labii superioris; 13 = zygomaticus minor; 14 = zygomaticus major; 15 = levator anguli oris; 16 = facial vein; 17 = facial artery; 18 = superior labial artery; 19 = orbicularis oris; 20 = mentalis; 21 = depressor labii inferioris; 22 = depressor anguli oris; 23 = platysma; 24 = risorius; 25 = masseter; 26 = buccal branches of facial nerve; 27 = buccal fat pad; 28 = accessory parotid gland; 29 = parotid duct; 30 = transverse facial artery; 31 = zygomatic branches of facial nerve; 32 = zygomatic arch; 33 = temporal branches of facial nerve; 34 = deep part of parotid gland; 35 = superficial part of parotid gland; 36 = marginal mandibular branch of facial nerve; 37 = cervical branch of facial nerve; 38 = external jugular vein; 39 = great auricular nerve; 40 = sternocleidomastoid; 41 = lesser occipital nerve; 42 = greater occipital nerve; 43 = occipital artery; 44 = occipital belly of occipitofrontalis; 45 = occipital vein.

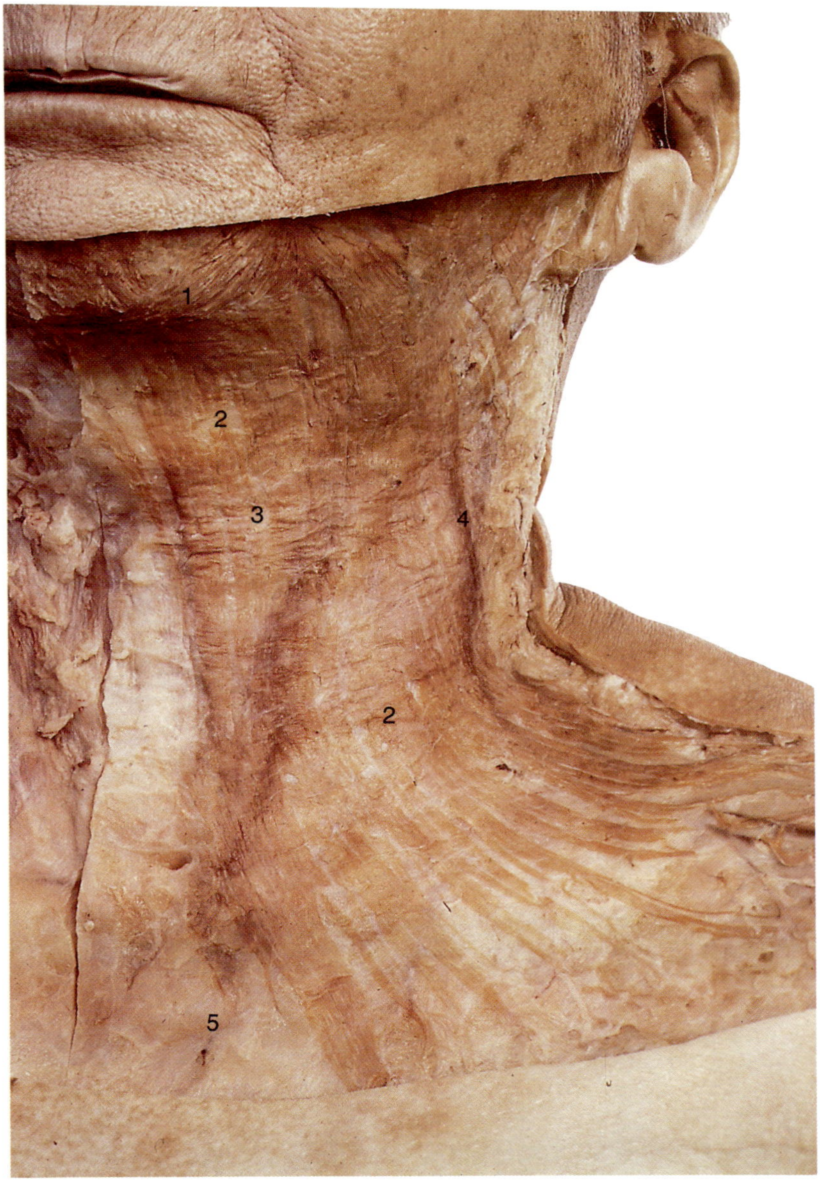

Figure 1–4. SMAS rhytidectomy: The platysma muscle. 1 = lower border of body of mandible; 2 = platysma; 3 = anterior jugular vein; 4 = external jugular vein; 5 = clavicle.

which are almost always clearly visible through the deep fascia of the head at surgery. The branches of the facial nerve enter the muscles on the deep surface, which permits a safe SMAS elevation. The relationship of the great auricular nerve to the sternomastoid muscle is also shown (see Figs. 1–3 and 1–5).

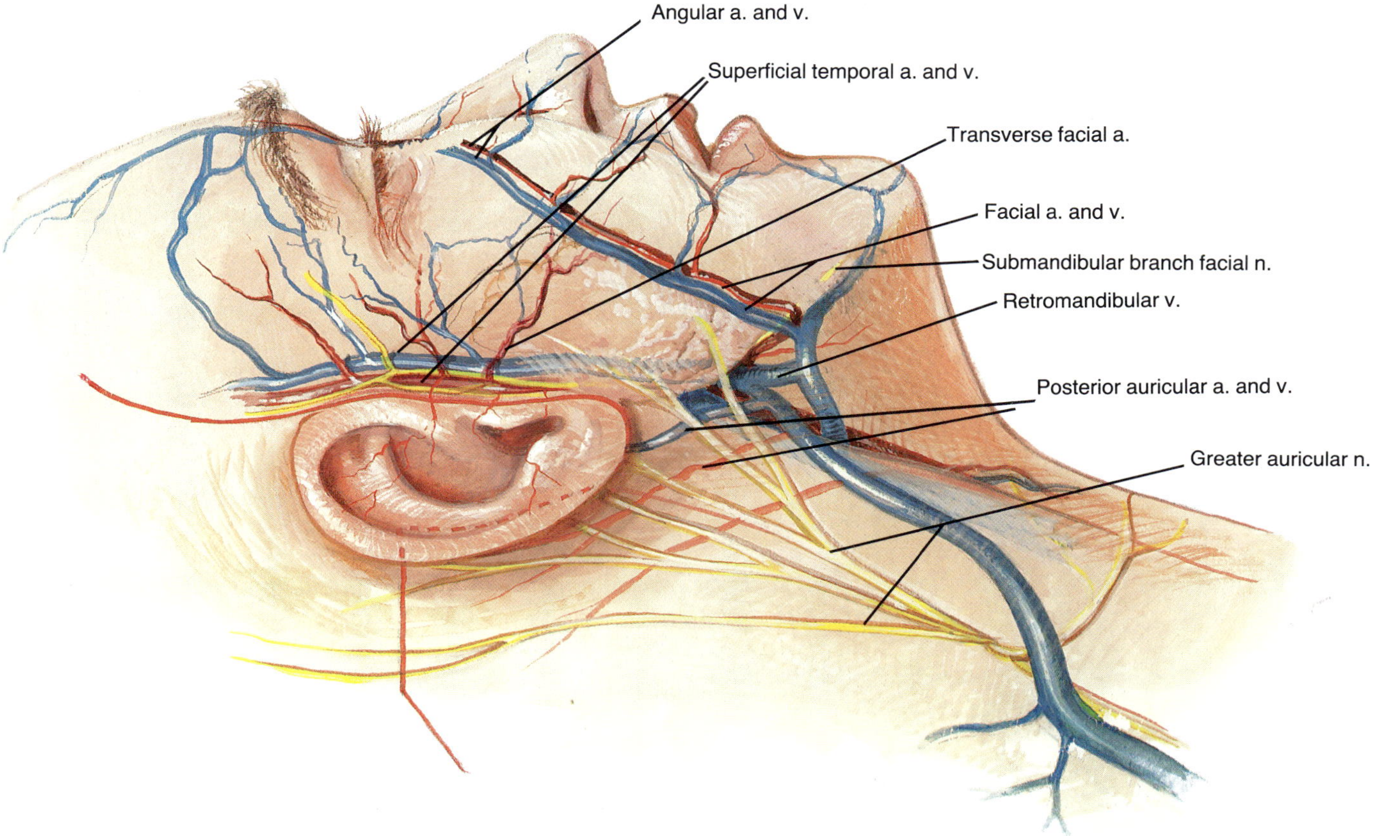

Figure 1–5. SMAS rhytidectomy: The blood vessels of the face and neck.

The Superficial Musculoaponeurotic System

Skoog[3] used the superficial fascia of the face clinically for a rhytidectomy technique, which was the first real change in the principal technique (subcutaneous) of face-lifting since its inception. This complex morphological unit is composed of skin, subcutaneous fat, and the superficial fascia, which could be elevated and advanced without skin undermining of the face. But it remained for Mitz and Peyronie[4] (1976) to describe this unit of anatomy of the face—the superficial musculoaponeurotic system. This classic paper stated the following:

1. The SMAS in the parotid and cheek areas is always present.
2. The subcutaneous fat of the cheek is divided into two layers by the SMAS.
3. Superficial to the SMAS, fat lobules are enclosed by fibrous septa which connect the SMAS with the dermis.
4. The SMAS of the cheek is continuous with the frontalis muscle superiorly and the platysma muscle inferiorly.
5. In the parotid area the fascia is thick, and in the cheek (masseter) area the fascia is thin.
6. The parotid (deep) fascia and SMAS are adherent in the pretragal area anteriorly for 1 to 2 cm.
7. The SMAS covers the superficial facial muscles and provides the attachment of the muscles to the dermis.
8. The branches of the anterior cervical plexus are located between the SMAS and the dermis.
9. The facial artery and vein are deep to the SMAS and send perforating branches through the SMAS.
10. The SMAS passes over the external surface of the zygoma to the temporal area (superficial temporal fascia).
11. The frontal branch of the facial nerve is deep to the SMAS.
12. The extent of the SMAS ranges from the mastoid (sternomastoid muscle) to the nasolabial fold in the anterior-posterior dimension and from the superficial temporal fascia to the platysma muscle in the superior-inferior dimension.
13. Tension on the SMAS is maintained superiorly by the frontalis muscle and the orbicularis oculi muscle and inferiorly by the platysma muscle.
14. The SMAS amplifies muscle contraction of the face as the posterior attachments (mastoid and pretragal) are stable and tension is varied in the temporal and platysma muscle region.

Mitz and Peyronie[4] suggested that surgical correction of aging changes resulting from the loss of elasticity of the SMAS could be better corrected by operating in a plane deep to the SMAS. This preserves the fibrous septum transmission of the contraction of the superficial facial muscles.

The SMAS in the temporal region presents as the superficial temporal fascia (temporoparietal fascia). It fuses superiorly (cephalad) with the galea, anteriorly with the frontalis muscle, and posteriorly with the occipitalis muscle. Inferiorly (caudad) it crosses the zygomatic arch to join the SMAS of the cheek. The temporal (frontal) branch of the facial nerve and superficial temporal artery and vein lie within the superficial temporal fascia. Stuzin and colleagues[5] demonstrated "that the nerve always travels in an anatomically predictable and constant plane." To protect the frontal branch, the dissection superior to the zygoma is deep to the superficial (temporoparietal) fascia and below the zygoma in the subcutaneous plane. The subcutaneous dissection usually overlaps the inferior extent of the superficial temporal (temporoparietal) fascia elevation (see Chapter 4, Fig. 4–1). The intervening tissue can be mobilized to a degree sufficient to advance the temporal skin and reduce the skin "swags" produced by a marked cheek advancement at the level of the outer canthus.

The Deep (Investing) Fascia of The Head And Neck[6]

Cephalad and ventrad to the hyoid bone, the superficial, or anterior layer of the deep fascia of the head and neck divides and embeds the submandibular gland. There is no distinct capsule of the submandibular gland as septa from the gland fuse with the anterior layer of the deep fascia. Cephalad and posterior to the submandibular gland, the investing, or deep fascia thickens and is attached to the inferior margin of the mandible. In the parotid region, it again splits into two laminae to incorporate the parotid gland in the same fashion as the submandibular gland. Above (cephalad) the parotid gland, the external layer of the deep fascia attaches to the zygoma and the deep layer to the temporal bone.

In the anterior triangle of the neck, the two layers of the deep fascia form a single layer. Just above and at the midportion of the clavicle, the external jugular vein perforates the superficial layer of the deep fascia, and is deep to the platysma (Fig. 1–5).

Below the hyoid bone and ventrally, the anterior, or superficial layer of the deep fascia splits and encloses the sternocleidomastoid muscle and the strap muscles of the neck.

The Facial Nerve (VII)

The branches of the facial nerve (see Fig. 1–3) are deep to the investing, or deep fascia of the head and neck except for the temporal, or frontal branch, which lies in the superficial temporal fascia, a continuation of the SMAS. In the parotid region, the deep and superficial fasciae are dense, thicker, and stronger. The facial nerve is protected by the deep fascia and encompassed by the parotid gland. Anterior, or medial to the parotid gland, the deep fascia over the superficial surface of the masseter muscle and the fat pad of Bichat is quite thin and fibers of the facial nerve branches are visible coursing through the area. The superficial fascia (SMAS) and the deep fascia are very adherent in the region of Bichat's fat pad. Though the facial nerve in this region is deep to the deep fascia, the deep fascia's thinness combined with the tightly adherent superficial (SMAS) and deep fasciae requires careful and patient dissection to separate the two layers.

The marginal mandibular branch of the facial nerve, a solitary branch, courses along the body of the mandible, but drops below the inferior mandibular border of the mandible approximately 1.0 cm or less (see Fig. 1–2) 19% of the time.[7] When the mandibular branch drops below the mandibular border, it recrosses the mandibular border at a more superficial level anterior to the facial artery to supply the quadratus labii inferioris and mentalis muscles on their superficial surface, rather than on the deep surface. The branch is seldom observed because the deep fascia is well developed, and the superficial and deep fascia plane is loosely adherent.

The cervical branch of the facial nerve penetrates the undersurface of the platysma muscle usually about 2.0 to 3.0 cm anterior to the posterior border of the platysma muscle approximately 0.5 to 2.0 cm below the inferior border of the mandible. A plexus of nerve fibers on the deep surface supplies the platysma muscle.

The Retaining Ligaments of the Face

Two types of retaining ligaments of the skin of the face have been described: osteocutaneous and fasciacutaneous ligaments.[8,9] It is possible these ligaments lend support to the face, or could as fixed or relatively fixed points, act to expand the range of facial expression possible by the mimetic muscles alone. That is, the retaining ligaments by their nature provide fixed, or pivot points, which upon contraction of the mimetic muscles magnify the range of facial expression.

The osteocutaneous retaining ligaments are the zygomatic and mandibular ligaments. These are stout fibrous attachments between the bone periosteum and the dermis.[8] The zygomatic ligament originates just behind the origin of the zygomaticus minor muscle on the inferior border of the zygomatic arch, and extends to the dermis. Furnas described bundles of white, firm fibers 3 mm in width and 0.5 mm in thickness, about 6 to 8 mm long, located 4.5 cm in front (anterior) of the tragus and containing an artery and a sensory nerve. Directly beneath the ligament there is an upper ramus of the zygomatic branch of the facial nerve. While Furnas pointed out that the ligament was not identifiable in 10% of the patients intraoperatively, this area is invariably a strong fibrous attachment that must be released.

In his original description of a sub-SMAS rhytidectomy, Skoog[3] pointed out the firm attachments in this area and the difficulty of the dissection in the area. If the release of this dense adherent area is not complete, the SMAS is not mobilized adequately in its upper (malar) portion.

The zygomatic ligament maintains the suspension of the soft tissue of the malar region, which along with the intervening tissues maintains a smooth or soft nasolabial fold. With attenuation of this osteocutaneous ligament and the intervening tissues, the perception is that the nasolabial fold is deepening, but in reality the excess soft tissue is rolling over the fixed line of the nasolabial crease.

The mandibular osteocutaneous ligament is a series of parallel, linear fibers that originate from about 1 cm above the lower border of the mandible in its anterior third. The ligament is about 4 to 5 mm long, contains a sensory nerve and a cutaneous artery, and attaches to the skin. The fibers also interdigitate with the platysma and triangularis muscles. Furnas[8] pointed out that this attachment inhibits the "lifting" force of the face-lift to the submandibular region and to the jowl area.

The parotid cutaneous support, or retaining ligament[9] is formed by a dense thickening of the superficial (SMAS) and deep fasciae of the head in the region of the parotid gland. Sharp dissection is necessary to separate this layer. The thickness and strength of the coalesced area seem to indicate there has been little attenuation of the parotid (deep) and superficial fasciae of the area. At operation, as this is a strong coalescence of superficial and deep fasciae, it can be retained intact, and utilized for the anchoring of the loose soft flexible tissues of the SMAS medial, or anterior, to the parotid region. Also, if the sub-SMAS plane of dissection is entered anterior to this dense coalescence of fascia, the areolar tissue between the SMAS and the deep fascia can be more easily separated anterior to the parotid gland. A more medial entrance to the sub-SMAS plane reduces the length of the SMAS to be advanced, or put another way, provides a stronger lifting force and fascia repair more proximate to the area to be restored.

Stuzin and colleagues[9] pointed out that in the area of the anterior border of the masseter muscle along with two other areas (along the zygomatic arch and overlying the parotid gland), the superficial and deep fasciae are very adherent as opposed to the areolar plane seen at the interface of the SMAS and the deep fascia in all other areas of the head and neck. Furnas[8] described this area anterior (medial) to the masseter muscle as the platysma cutaneous ligament, but Stuzin and colleagues[9] believed that the fibers of this adherent area extending along the anterior border of the masseter from the malar region to the border of the mandible originate from the masseter muscle and extend vertically to the cutaneous layer. They believed attenuation of this masseteric cutaneous ligament with aging in association with tethering from mandibular ligaments results in delineation of the borders of jowl formation.

Skoog,[3] in his classic description of sub-SMAS rhytidectomy, managed this adherent area anterior (medial) to the anterior border of the masseter muscle and the fat pad of Bichat by penetrating the area with closed scissors and upon spreading of the blades, bluntly released the tissues to the nasolabial fold area and its extension caudad to the oral commissure. Intraoperatively, these bands of condensed connective tissue can be transected sufficiently to obtain a more complete release of the tissues. Whether sub-SMAS, or supra-SMAS as noted by Furnas, this is an area of indistinct tissue planes without clear landmarks, and orientation can be difficult.

The Mimetic Muscles of the Face

Freilinger and coauthors[10] described the surgical anatomy of the mimic muscle system and considered the three-dimensional aspects of four layers of facial muscle. The most superficial layer includes the orbicularis oculi, the superficial portion of the zygomaticus minor, and the depressor anguli oris. The second layer contains the platysma, the risorius, the zygomaticus major, the deeper portion of the zygomaticus minor, and the levator labii superioris alaeque nasi. The third layer consists of the levator labii superioris and the orbicularis oris, and the fourth layer consists of the levator angularis oris, the mentalis, and the buccinator. The peripheral branches of the facial nerve supply the first three layers on the deep side of the muscle. In addition to protecting the nerve, the muscle layering of the mimetic muscles is extremely significant in the malar region of a SMAS rhytidectomy because it is necessary to change the plane of dissection from sub-SMAS to a more superficial (subcutaneous) level.

After the adherent retaining ligament of the zygomatic area is released, the lower border of the orbicularis oculi muscle is elevated superiorly in the direction of the inferior orbital rim. Proceeding inferiorly (caudad) with the separation of the superficial (SMAS) from the deep fascia, the sub-SMAS plane of dissection is deep to the zygomaticus major muscle. (Freilinger and coauthors also described a ramus of the zygomatic branch of the facial nerve, which crosses over the zygomaticus major muscle in its superior third on its superficial surface to reach the inferior part of the orbicularis oculi.) At the lateral border of the zygomaticus major muscle, the SMAS is penetrated medially, which moves the dissection from a sub-SMAS to a superficial SMAS (subcutaneous) level[2] (see Fig. 5–1). The dissection anterior (medial) to the lateral border of the zygomaticus major muscle is subcutaneous (see Fig. 1–2). Except for the orbicularis oculi, the mimetic muscles of the SMAS are eliminated from the elevation of the SMAS in the region of the zygomatic muscles. As there are no major mimetic muscle attachments to the skin in the area, fibrous septa interruption described by Mitz and Peyronie[4] is not a factor.

The Blood Supply of the Face

The blood supply in a rhytidectomy of the face originates from the external carotid artery (see Fig. 1–5). The facial, labial, and angular arteries in the medial area of the face and the superficial temporal artery in the lateral face, or preauricular region frame the operative site of the SMAS-platysma facelift. Inside the frame, or between the borders of these major vessels, the surgeon encounters the perforating vessels of the transverse facial artery and submental artery. The postauricular skin is supplied by the posterior auricular branch of the external carotid artery.

Whetzel and Mathes,[11] in a comprehensive study of the arterial anatomy of the face with ink and blue latex injection techniques in fresh cadavers, defined the perforating branches of the transverse facial and submental arteries. They divided the cutaneous blood supply of the face into musculocutaneous (anterior area of the face), fasciacutaneous (lateral area of the face), and a thin, deep fasciacutaneous circulation. Their work revealed that the perforator arteries of the transverse facial artery "pass directly through the SMAS and subcutaneous tissue without branching to arborize extensively in the subdermis." In the majority of cases studied, the transverse facial artery had only a single large perforator penetrating the SMAS. As well, the submental artery area most often had only a single perforator. Upon reaching the subdermal plexus, the transverse facial artery perforators develop large and long terminal branches. The submental perforators branched three or four times to supply separate areas of the dermis. By measuring from bone landmarks, the site of the transverse facial artery perforator was predictable within 2+ cm 95% of the time. The submental perforator (as well as others in the study) was much less predictable. The transverse facial artery perforators covered an area of 6.0 by 7.0 cm, with the borders anteriorly in line with the inner canthus, posteriorly 1.5 cm anterior to the auditory canal, superiorly 1.5 cm above the zygomatic arch, and inferiorly 1 cm below the oral commissure. The area covered by the submental artery measured 5.0 by 5.0 cm, with borders anteriorly 1.5 cm lateral to the oral commissure, posteriorly 2 cm anterior to the sternomastoid muscle, superiorly adjacent to the transverse facial artery section, and inferiorly 3 cm below the mandibular border.

The anterior, or medial area of the face is supplied by the facial artery and its branches, the inferior and superior labial arteries, and the angular branch lateral to the nose. The facial artery appears from under the mandible (deep to the submandibular gland) at approximately the anterior border of the masseter muscle. It is deep to the platysma, risorius, and zygomaticus major and minor muscles, and lies superficial to the buccinator and levator anguli oris muscles. Hollinshead[6] stated that it gives off "twigs" to the masseter muscle and unnamed branches that anastomose with the other arteries that reach the face. Whetzel and Mathes[11] described a deep plexus of small vessels that communicates with the subdermal plexus through a dense population of small musculocutaneous arteries. The vessels of this musculocutaneous region (anterior, or medial area of the face) and the fasciacutaneous region (lateral, or posterior area of the face–SMAS) approximate each other lateral to the nasolabial fold.

Whetzel and Mathes[11] also pointed out that sub-SMAS dissection with transection of the lateral fasciacutaneous perforators, which places the origin of the blood supply of the flap on the anterior musculocutaneous perforators, would not be expected to increase the blood supply to the flap.

In the scalp and postauricular region, the deep fascial layer and the subdermal layer are close together. The superficial temporal artery in the temporoparietal fascia and the posterior auricular artery supply the perforators in these areas.[11]

References

1. McMinn, R.M.H., Hutchings, R.T., and Logan, B.M.: Color Atlas of Head and Neck Anatomy. Chicago, Year Book Medical Publishers, 1981, pp. 92, 112, 118.
2. Barton, F.E., Jr.: The SMAS and nasolabial fold. Plast. Reconstr. Surg. 1992; 89:1054–1059.
3. Skoog, T.: Plastic Surgery—New Methods. Philadelphia, W.B. Saunders, 1974, pp. 300–330.
4. Mitz, V. and Peyronie, M.: The superficial musculoaponeurotic system (SMAS) in the parotid and cheek area. Plast. Reconstr. Surg. 1976; 58:80–88.
5. Stuzin, J.M., Wagstrom, L., Kowomoto, H.K., and Wolfe, S.A.: Anatomy of the frontal branch of the facial nerve: The significance of the temporal fat pad. Plast. Reconstr. Surg. 1989; 89:441–451.
6. Hollinshead, W.H. Anatomy for Surgeons, The Head and Neck, ed. 2. Hagerstown, MD, Harper and Row, 1968, pp. 309–329, 331–367.
7. Dingman, R.O. and Grabb, W.C.: Surgical anatomy of the mandibular ramus of the facial nerve based on the dissection of 100 facial halves. Plast. Reconstr. Surg. 1962; 29:266–272.
8. Furnas, D.W.: The retaining ligaments of the cheek. Plast. Reconstr. Surg. 1989; 83:11–16.
9. Stuzin, J.M., Baker, T.J., and Gordon, H.L.: The relationship of the superficial and deep fascias: Relevance to rhytidectomy and aging. Plast. Reconstr. Surg. 1992; 89:441–451.
10. Freilinger, G., Gruber, H., Happak, W., and Pechmann, U.: Surgical anatomy of the mimic muscle system and the facial nerve: Importance for reconstructive and aesthetic surgery. Plast. Reconstr. Surg. 1987; 80:686–690.
11. Whetzel, T.P. and Mathes, S.J.: Arterial anatomy of the face: An analysis of vascular territories and perforating cutaneous vessels. Plast. Reconstr. Surg. 1992; 89:591–605.

TWO

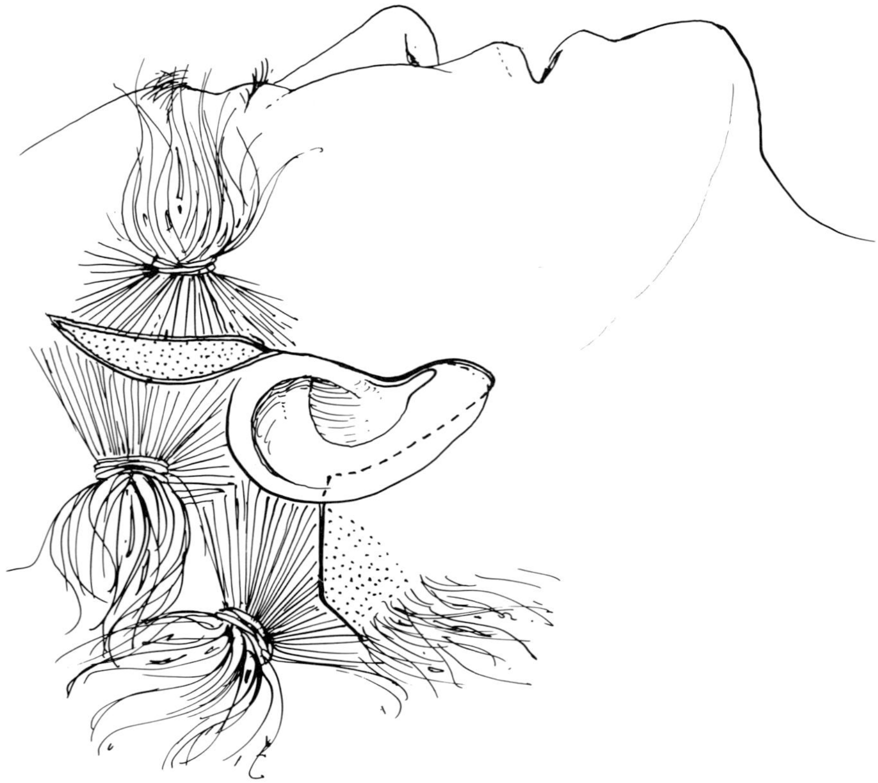

The Preparation of the Operative Field and Skin Markings of the Incisions

Prior to the planning and placing of the skin markings, a general anesthetic is administered. The skin markings of the incisions are applied. The hair in the temporal and occipital regions is shaved in the operative area and the remaining hair is held away from the incision lines with rubber bands in the adjacent hair. A local anesthesia with a high dilution of epinephrine is injected in the initial operative area. The preparation of the hair, the skin markings, and the infiltration of an anesthetic solution into the initial operative site are completed (Fig. 2–1). The head and neck can now be prepared and draped as a sterile "clean" field. The details of the preoperative preparation follow.

Marking the Temporal Area Incisions

Redundant temporal scalp is pressed into a fold to estimate the amount of scalp to be removed in this area (Fig. 2–2). The borders of the fold are outlined utilizing a sharpened applicator stick (wood) and 1% methylene blue solution (sterile)* (or the reader's choice of marking technique). (All mention of marking that follows uses this technique.) At wound closing, further excision for hairline (sideburn) adjustment and removal of sufficient redundant tissue may be necessary.

The Preauricular Incision Marking

The estimated amount of redundant skin of the temporal region to be removed has been outlined. The preauricular skin marking (see Fig. 2–1) follows; the mark is placed at the skin crease formed by the attachment of the

*1% Methylene blue (sterile, 10cc ampule), American Regent Laboratories, Inc., Shirley, NY 11967.

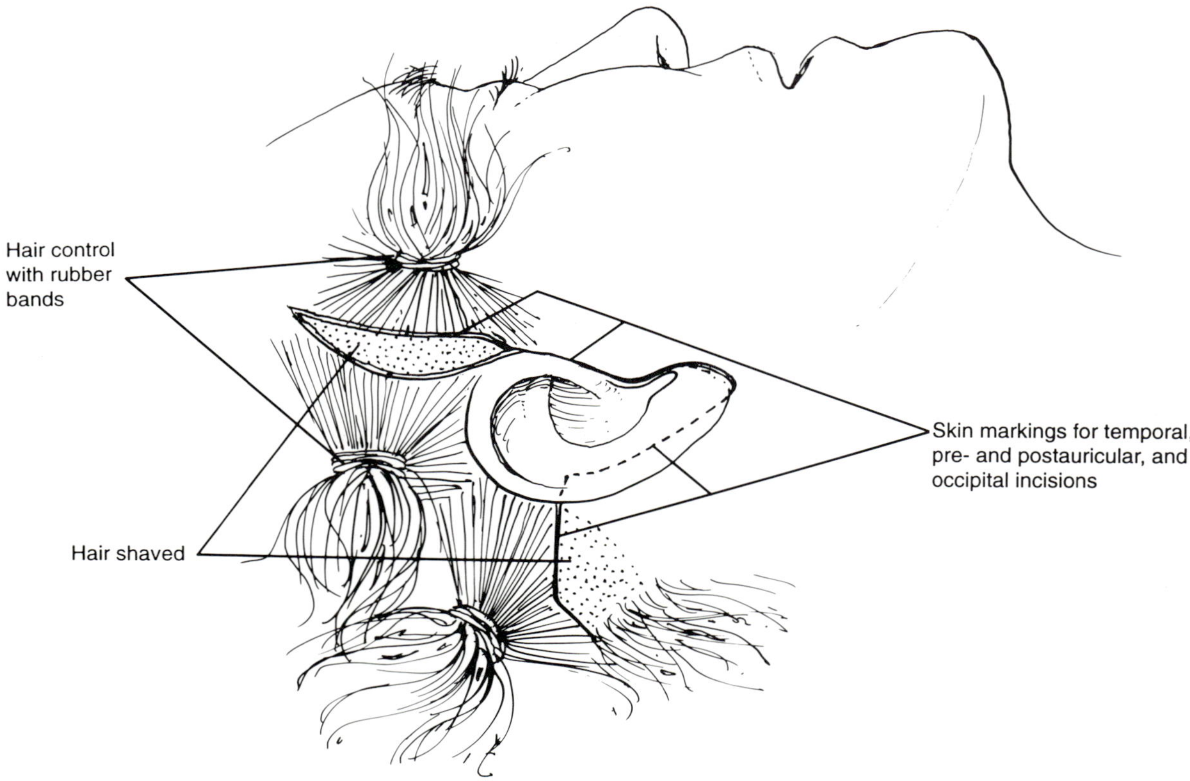

A

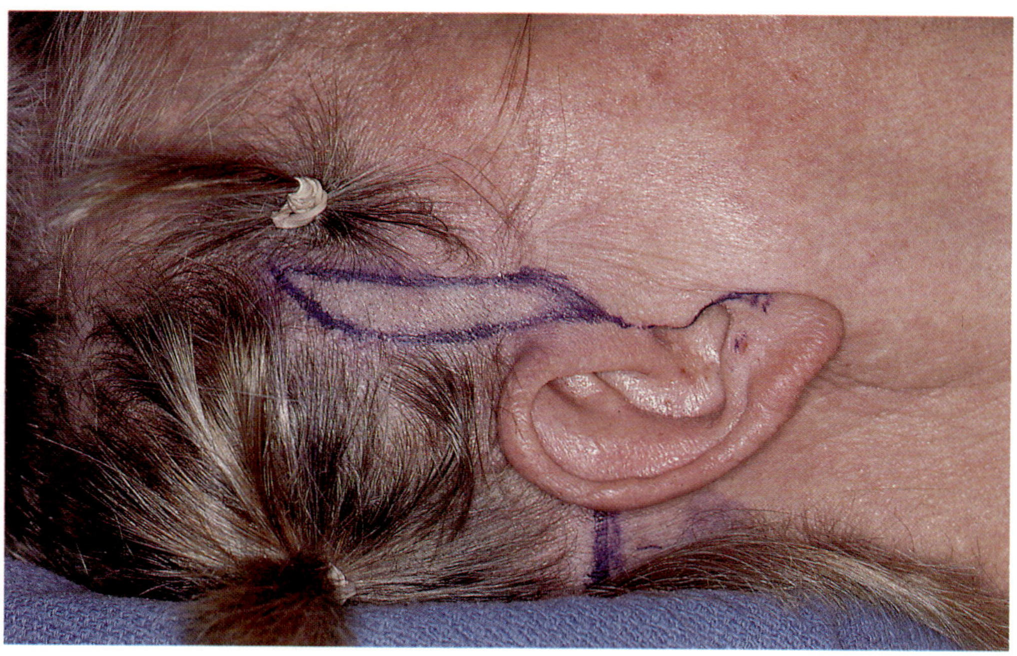

B

Figure 2–1. SMAS rhytidectomy: Hair and scalp preparation; skin incisions marked. **A.** Illustration of the intraoperative photograph (B). **B.** Intraoperative photograph of a patient with the hair prepared and with the skin incision markings of the temporal, the preauricular (and the tragal), the postauricular and the occipital regions applied.

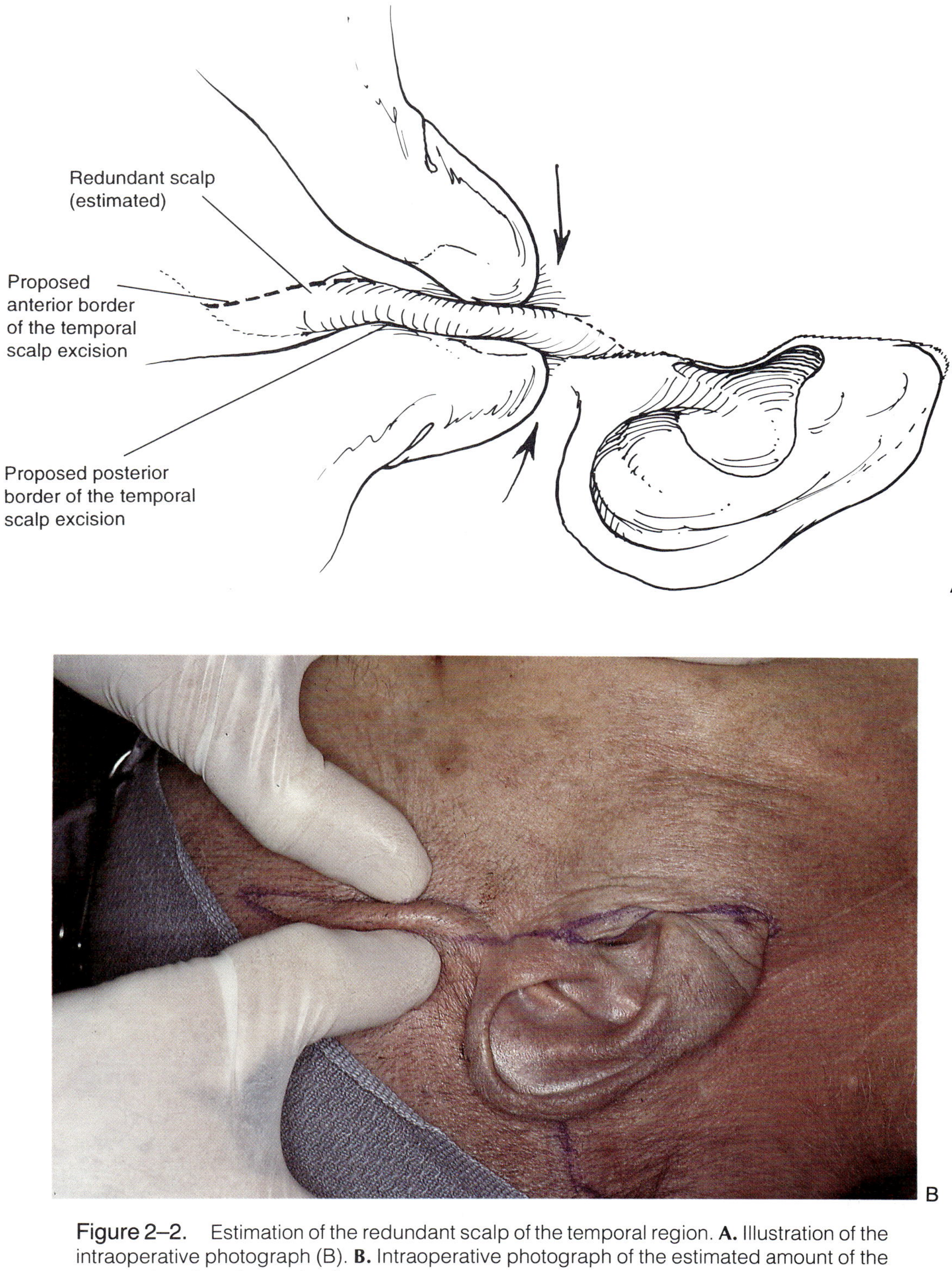

A

B

Figure 2–2. Estimation of the redundant scalp of the temporal region. **A.** Illustration of the intraoperative photograph (B). **B.** Intraoperative photograph of the estimated amount of the temporal scalp to be excised.

helix to the skull. Either a pretragal or tragus rim incision is outlined (Fig. 2–3). The line of incision, whether it emerges from the tragal notch or is pretragal, continues in the skin crease of the lobule of the ear created by the attachment of the lobule to the skin of the cheek (see Fig. 2–1A).

The Choice of a Tragus or Preauricular Incision

The choice as to which incision to utilize in the tragus region depends on the anatomy involved, the patient's desires, and/or the surgeon's preference. While anatomy probably should determine the choice, the latter reasons usually prevail.

Where the cheek skin is thin, the tragus skin usually will be thinner, and consequently the tragus will be sculptured and well defined. A tragus rim incision is ideal as it preserves the sculptured and chic appearance of the defined tragus and breaks up a continuous scar line in the pretragal area (see Fig. 2–3B).

In the patient with thick skin of the cheek and a less-defined tragus (due to the thicker skin extending over the tragus), and in whom the angle of the tragus with cheek is more vertical, the junction of the tragus with the cheek will create a crease (see Fig. 2–2B). If the incision is placed in the crease, the resultant minimal scar is rarely observed after healing is complete.

If the angle of the tragus with the cheek is flat or very obtuse and the skin over the tragus is thick, a tragus rim incision can be used as, in this case, the preauricular/pretragal crease is nonexistent or ill-defined (see Fig. 2–1B).

When the patient understands that superior results are achieved by adhering to the particular anatomy presented and known plastic surgery principles, usually a choice can be made based upon the anatomy.

However, there is no reason a tragus rim incision cannot be used in all cases. If it is used in all cases, the patient must understand clearly that if some of the factors mentioned are ignored, the results may not be as desirable.

The tragus rim incision follows the contour of the tragus and is placed just on the posterior border of the rim. It crosses the tragus notch of the ear on its anterior superior edge and forms a gentle curve, matching, when possible, the curvature of the attachment of the lobule of the ear. This assists (see Chapter 6, Figs. 6–10A and 6–12) in the prevention of a scar contracture and/or offset of the skin edges in the area of the scar extending from the tragal notch to the preauricular crease of the lobule of the ear. This creates somewhat of a lazy "s," which lengthens the scar. If somewhat of a lazy "s" is not incorporated, or the length of the scar is too short (too straight), a scar contracture and skin offset may occur. The appearance of this short scar creates the impression that the skin of the lower face is hanging from or held up by the tragus.

The preauricular incision is the incision of choice in the fatter individual, or the individual with a thicker subcutaneous fat layer, or so-called "heavy face," and a visually well-defined preauricular crease. Even if the preauricular crease is not well defined in a thick-skin individual, a preauricular incision preserves the normal appearance of the tragus. Again, if the angle of the

Figure 2–3. Pretragal and tragus rim incision markings. **A, B.** Illustration of a pretragal and tragal rim incision, respectively.

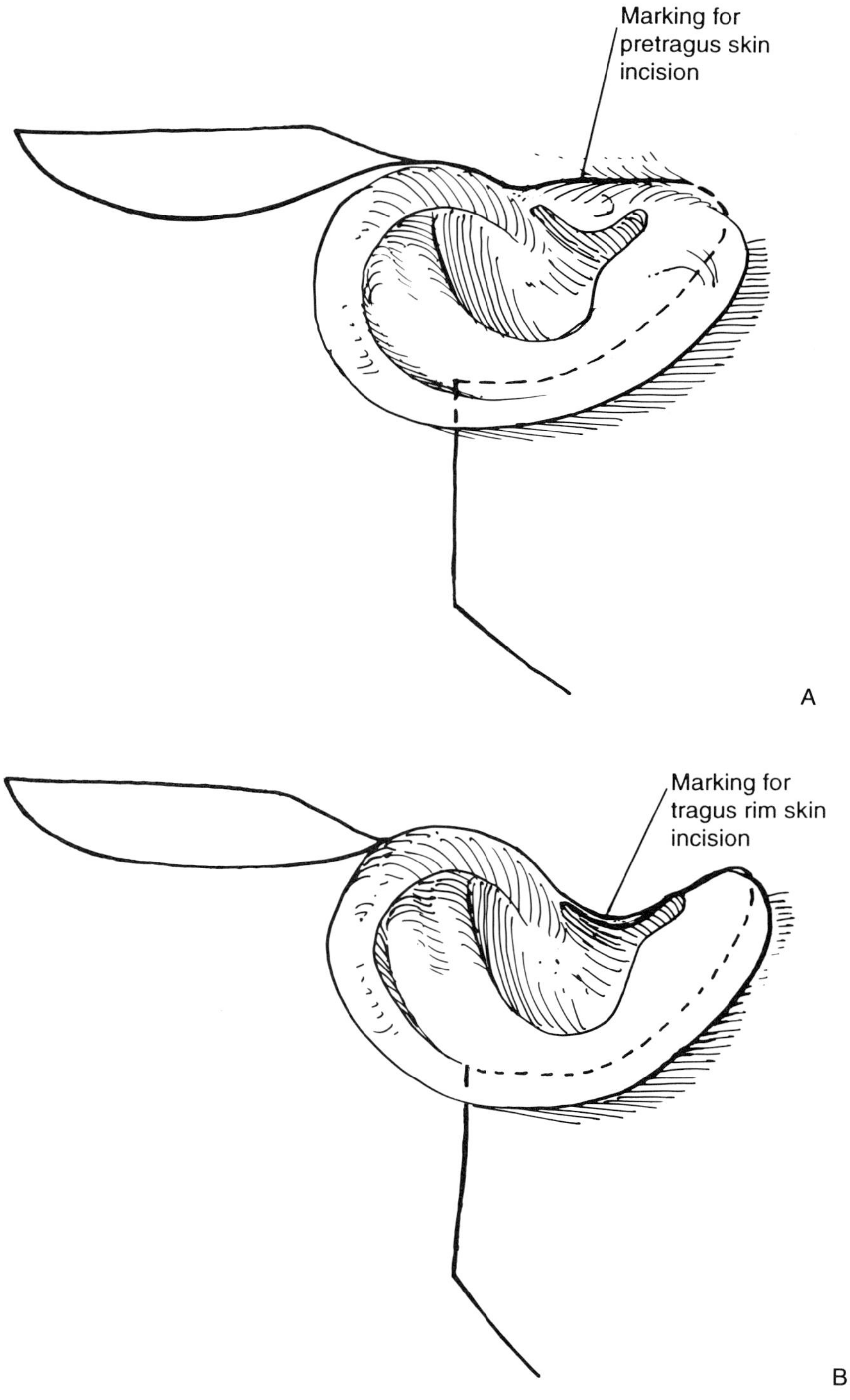

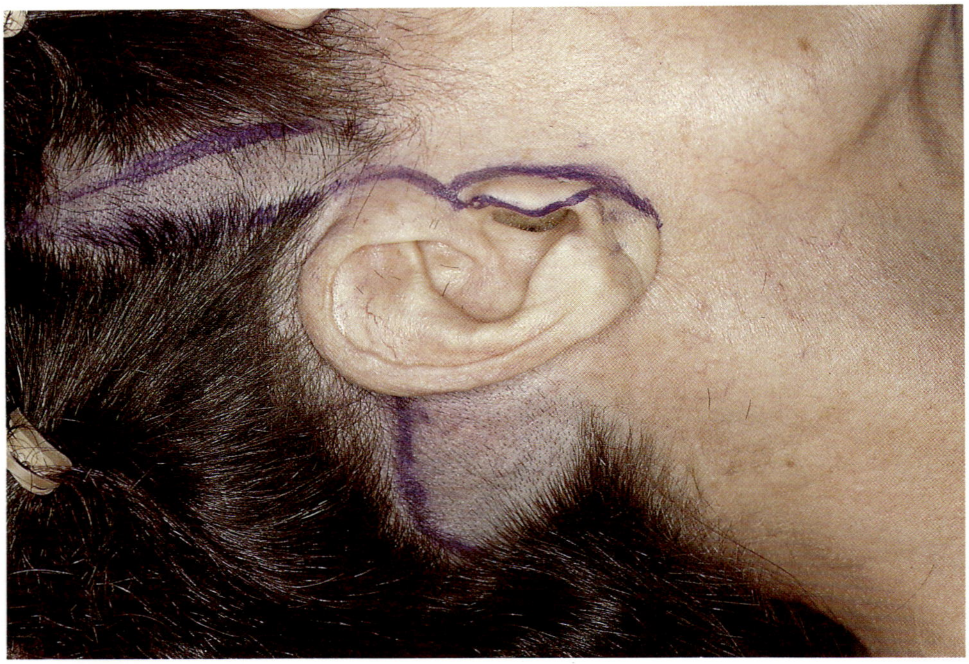

C

Figure 2–3 (continued) **C.** Intraoperative photograph of the pretragal and the tragal rim incisions applied.

tragus is flat or obtuse and the skin is thick, a rim incision can be utilized (see Fig. 2–1B).

The Postauricular and Occipital Incision Markings

The ear is elevated approximately to a vertical (90-degree) position to the head and the marking carried around the lobule approximately 1 mm below the crease of the lobule. At the level of the caudal border of the concha, the marking begins to angle up on the medial surface of the concha, and continues at this level to a point opposite (on a horizontal line) the junction of the inferior crus with the helix rim of the ear (Fig. 2–4). At this level the postauricular incision is approximately 4 to 5 mm above the postauricular sulcus.

At the level stated above, the occipital marking extends in a horizontal direction (or at a 90-degree angle from the temporal incision) (see Fig. 2–4). This places the occipital incision at a level of the greatest width of the ear, which normally will cover the non–hair-bearing area behind the ear. This produces the shortest possible exposed scar between the postauricular sulcus and the hairline. At a point just anterior to the occipital protuberance, the occipital marking is angled in a caudad direction. The length of the angled portion of the occipital incision is approximately 2.0 to 2.5 cm. When the skin of the neck in the occipital region is closed (see Chapter 6, Fig. 6–4), the angling of the incision permits the skin of the neck to be redraped at a different angle than the skin of the cheek. This provides the optimum posterior superior and lateral (posterior) advancement of the skin of the neck. Also, the angled portion of the incision assists in the prevention and/or

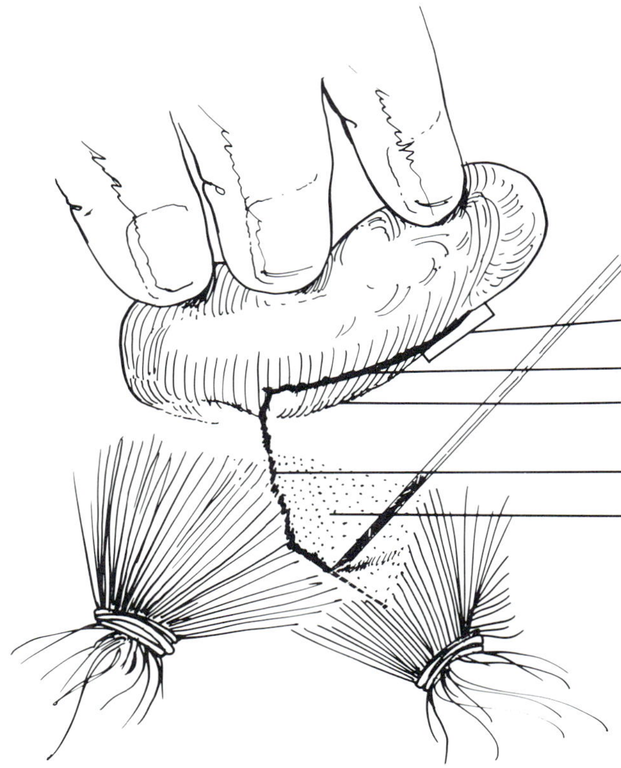

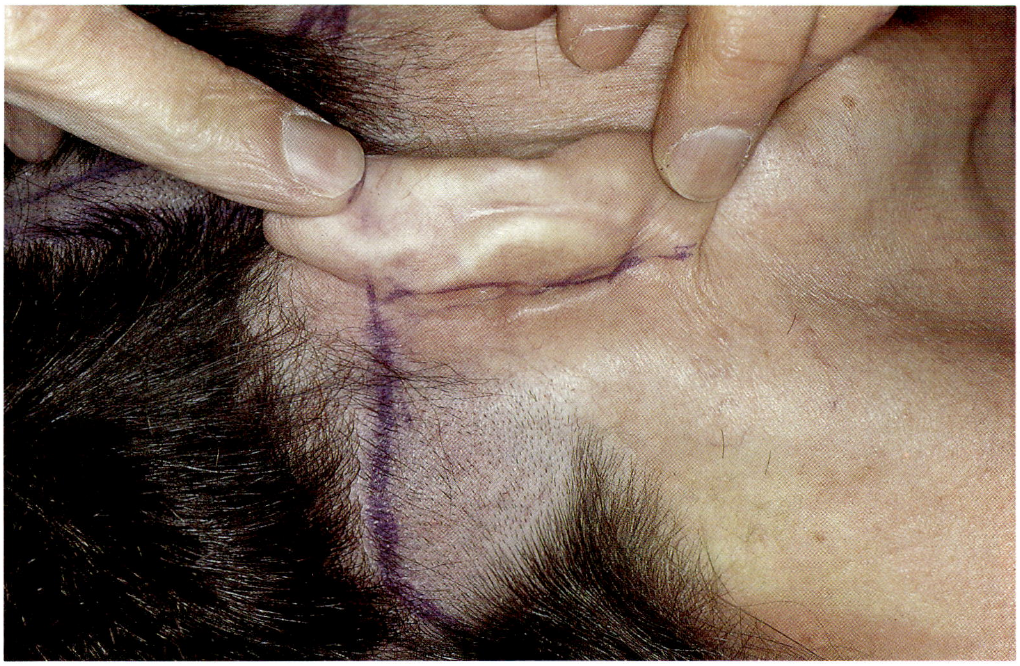

Figure 2–4. Postauricular and occipital skin markings. **A.** Illustration of photograph (B). **B.** Intraoperative photograph.

removal of a "dog-ear" of the scalp, which occurs at the terminal end of the occipital incision.[1]

Hair Preparation

The first step in hair preparation is being certain to inform the patient that the hair should not be set or styled prior to admission to the hospital. Second, if hair tinting or coloring is desired, it should be done several days prior to the date of surgery. Also, if tinting or coloring is not done preoperatively, it will be approximately 3 weeks postoperatively before it can be scheduled. Third, inform the patient that the hair will be washed the day of surgery with an antiseptic soap,* and that nothing is to be applied to the hair (spray, etc.) after the antiseptic-soap shampoo.

Probably one of the greatest concerns of the patient is how much hair will need to be cut to perform the surgery. The answer is only as much as necessary to place the incisions, and upon closure of the wounds, hair-bearing areas will be approximated and the head of hair will appear normal after surgery.

At the operating table and after the skin markings are applied, the hair over the temporal and the occipital incisions is cut and/or the area is shaved. The hair adjacent to the incisions in the scalp is bunched and a sterile elastic band (now "clean")** is applied. Usually only three or four groupings per side are needed to clear the hair adjacent to the incisions (see Fig. 2–1).

Anesthesia

General anesthesia is the method of choice. This method provides the best control of the patient's operative condition, and with the agents utilized today, the recovery is rapid. An anesthetist or anesthesiologist is employed to manage the details pertaining to the anesthesia (the pre-, intra- and post-operative period). The agents employed for the general anesthesia are the choice of the anesthetist or anesthesiologist.

The general anesthesia is administered prior to preparation of the hair. This has the advantage of a shorter preparation period and relieves the patient of further anxiety.

After the general anesthesia is administered and the skin markings are applied, and prior to hair and face preparation for a clean draping of the head, a long-acting local anesthetic (marcaine 0.25%***) with 1:400,000 or 1:600,000 epinephrine is prepared. (One ml of epinephrine 1:1000 dilution is diluted with 9 ml of saline. 1.5 ml of the 10 ml solution of epinephrine is added to 60 ml of marcaine 0.25% local anesthesia solution. The result is a 1:400,000 dilution of epinephrine in a slightly less than 0.25% marcaine solution.) Either of these concentrations of epinephrine provides sufficient

---

*Ultradex, 3% chloroxylenol, Dexide, Inc., Fort Worth, TX 76118.
**Office supply type sterilized.
***Marcaine 0.25% Winthrop Pharmaceutical, Inc., Division of Sterling Drug, NY, NY 10016.

vasoconstriction of the tissues without significant systemic effects. Initially, the submental and anterior cervical regions of the neck are infiltrated (Fig. 2–5) (approximately 10–15 ml). A 10 ml syringe with a 25 gauge 3 1/2 inch spinal needle attached is utilized to introduce the marcaine-epinephrine mixture into the subcutaneous tissue. Incision lines of the face (Fig. 2–6) and the cheek and the posterior cervical region of the right side of the face (Fig. 2–7) are infiltrated (approximately 20–25 ml) after the submental restoration is completed. When the right side of the face has been closed, the incision lines and the cheek and posterior cervical region on the left side are infiltrated.

The total volume of the marcaine/epinephrine solution injected over a period of one and a half hours is between 50–60 ml.

The local infiltration of the subcutaneous tissues of the cheeks need not extend medially from the preauricular area for a distance greater than 3.5 to 4.0 cm or the point of anticipated penetration and elevation of the SMAS. Skoog[2] pointed out that there is little bleeding at the sub-SMAS level when the compound morphological unit (SMAS subcutaneous fat and skin) is intact, except for a perforating artery and vein in the malar region.

The area medial (anterior) to the zygomaticus major muscle where the dissection becomes superficial to the SMAS in the subcutaneous fat should be infiltrated for the epinephrine effect (Fig. 2–7). Otherwise, one can expect considerable oozing from this rather inaccessible subcutaneous area.

After the general anesthesia is established, and the skin markings have been placed and the submental region and the anterior cervical areas, bilateral, are infiltrated with the marcaine-epinephrine solution, the head and neck are prepared with the same antiseptic soap utilized to wash the hair.

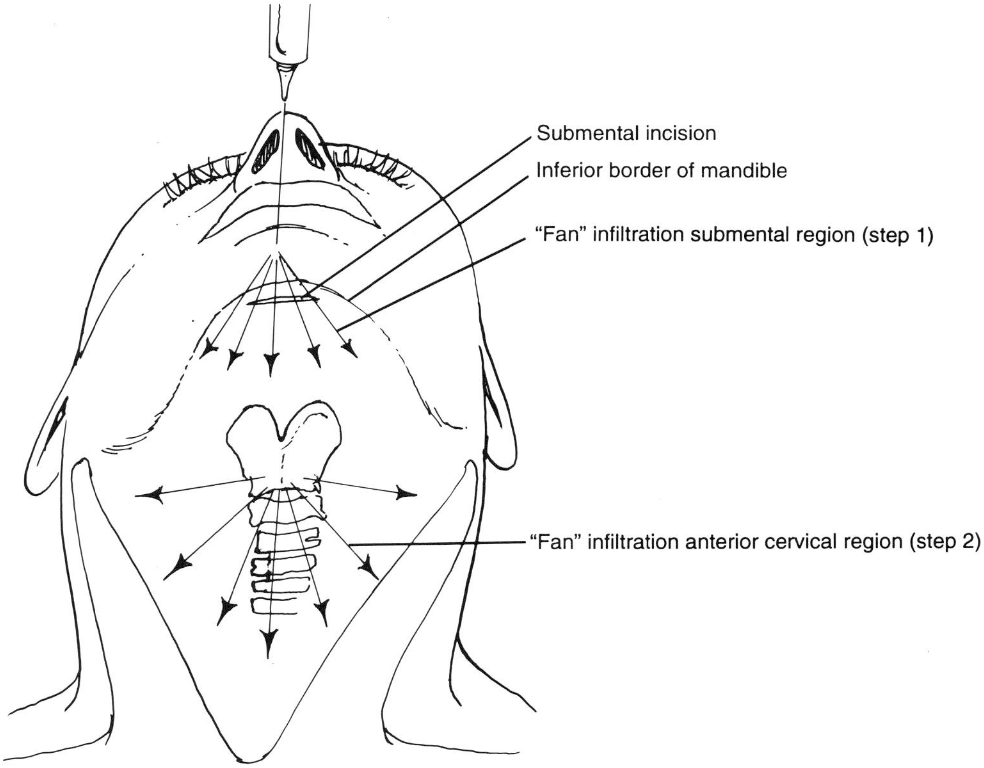

Figure 2–5. Local anesthesia/epinephrine infiltration of the submental region (step 1) and the anterior cervical region, bilaterally (step 2).

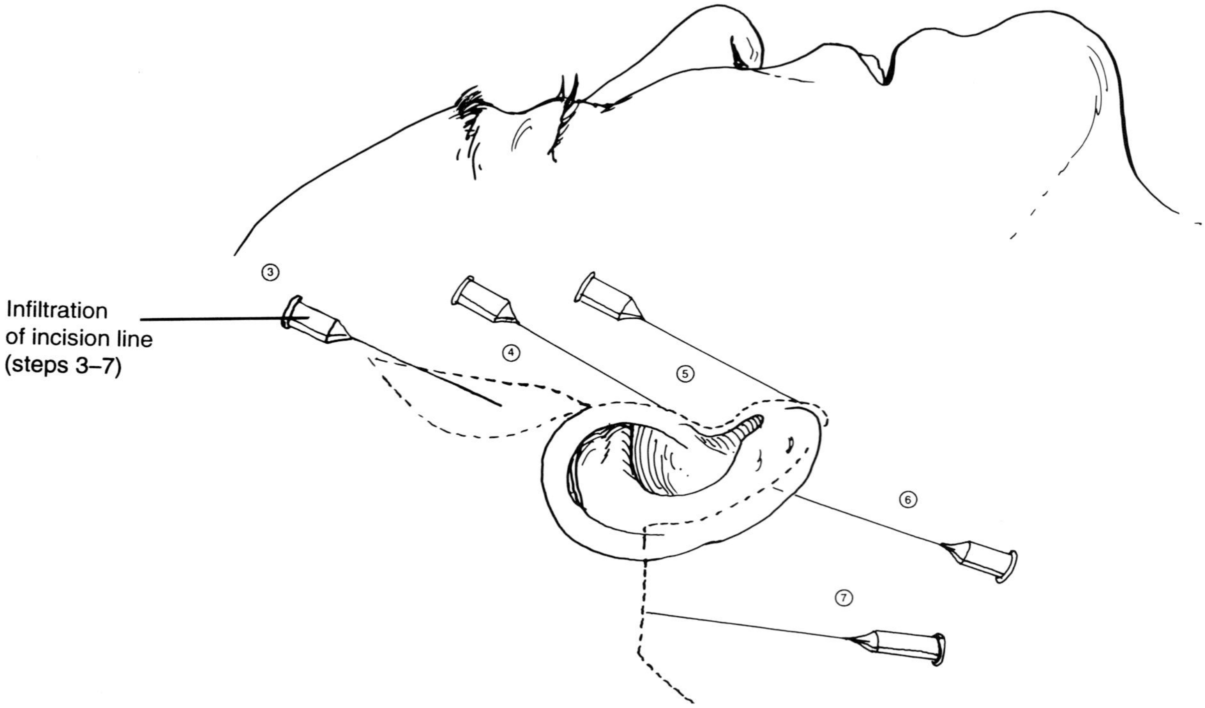

Figure 2–6. Local anesthesia/epinephrine infiltration of the skin incisions of the temporal, preauricular and postauricular, and occipital regions (steps 3–7).

Figure 2–7. Local anesthesia/epinephrine infiltration of the subcutaneous tissues of the temporal, zygomatic/infraorbital, preauricular and postauricular, occipital, and infraorbital regions.

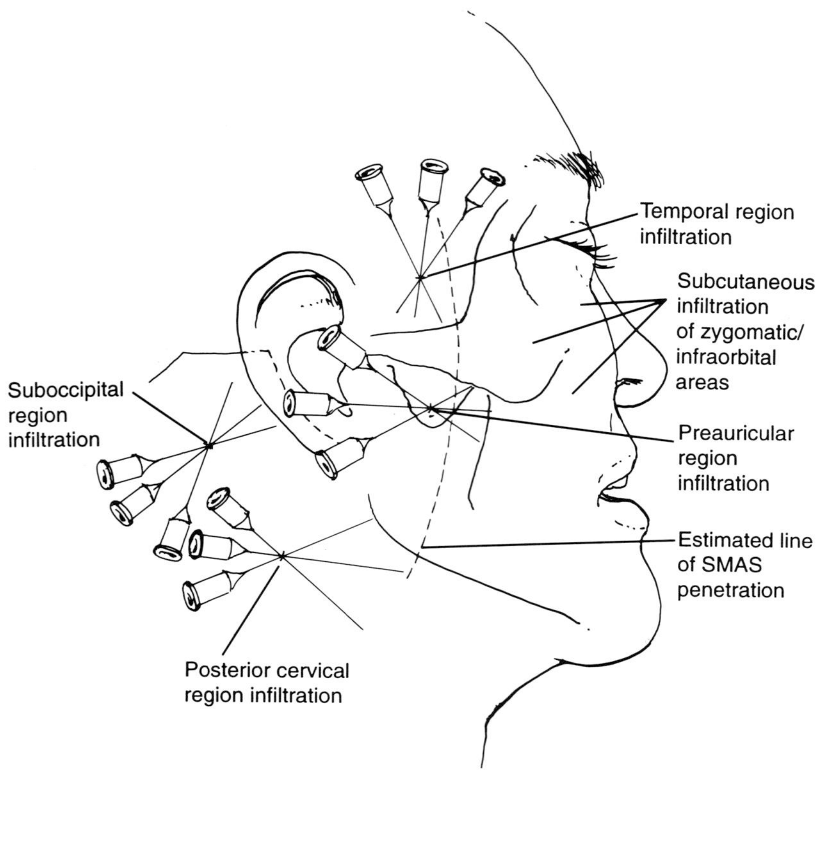

The anesthesia tubes are covered with a sterile clear drape,* and sterile towels are used to block out the sterile ("clean") field and to cover the hair.

While general anesthesia is preferable, face-lift surgery can be well managed utilizing local infiltration and/or regional nerve blocks in conjunction with various intravenous drugs for sedation or dissociation. These techniques require that a good respiratory exchange be maintained by an oral airway and a supplemental supply of oxygen be administered. Trained personnel should be in attendance as the surgeon's preoccupation with the surgery does not permit close monitoring of the patient's general condition.

The same technique of local infiltration of the neck and face is used as described when a general anesthetic is administered followed by local infiltration of the tissues as an epinephrine transport (see Figs. 2–5, 2–6, and 2–7). A long-acting local anesthetic agent (marcaine 0.25%) with a 1:400,000 or 1:600,000 dilution of epinephrine added to the solution is preferred.

A regional nerve block with infiltration of the incision lines is also a very satisfactory technique.[2] It has the advantages of saving some time in administration and of reducing tissue swelling and bruising of the face caused by infiltration of the tissues. Except for the pterygoid fossa instillation, the technique is easily performed and with practice the instillation in the pterygoid fossa becomes routine. A long-acting local anesthetic with the same

*Steri-drape (1000), 3M, Medical Surgical Division, St. Paul, Minnesota 55144.

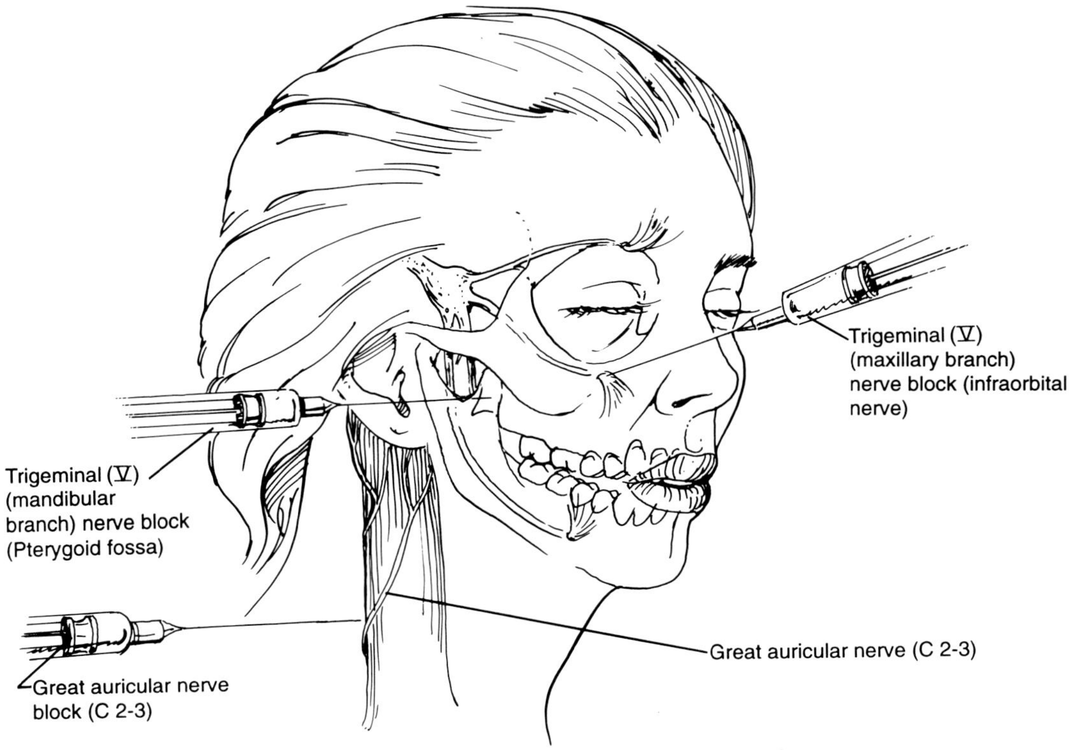

Figure 2–8. Regional nerve block of the infraorbital and mandibular branches of the trigeminal nerve (V) and the greater auricular nerve.

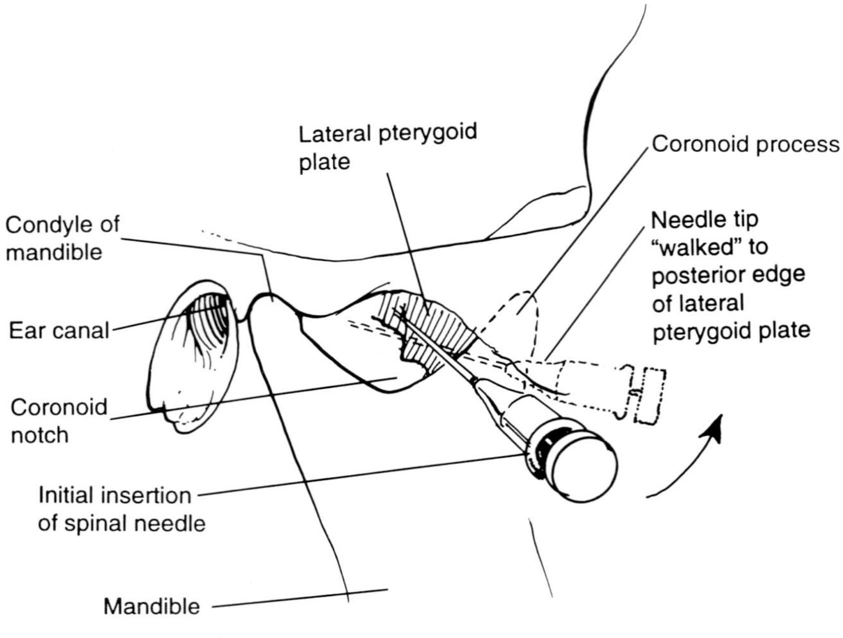

A. Lateral view of pterygoid fossa block technique

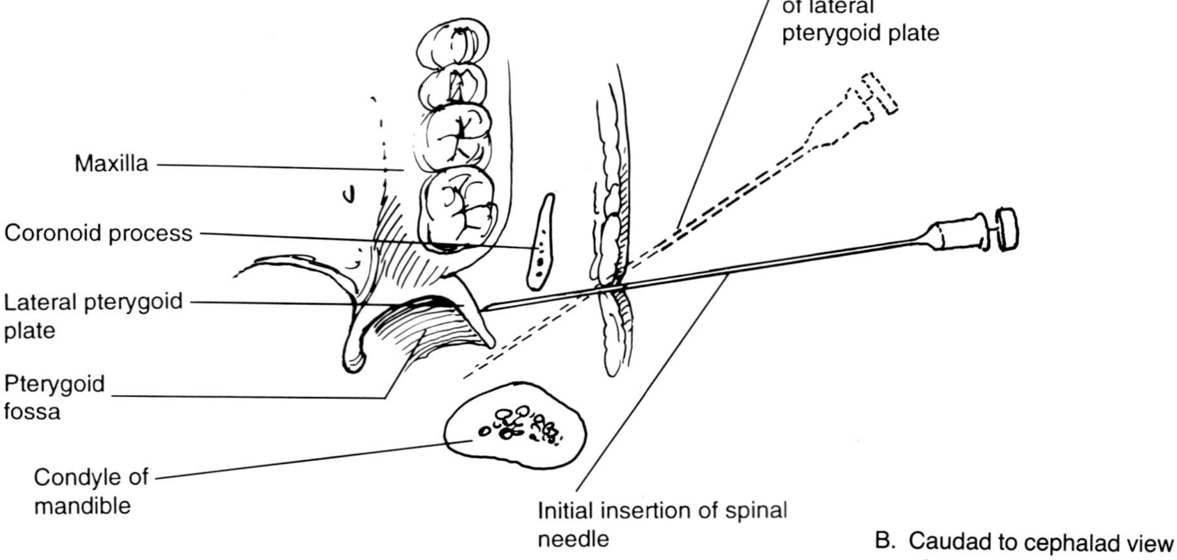

B. Caudad to cephalad view of pterygoid fossa block technique

Figure 2–9. Technique of the trigeminal nerve (V) (mandibular branch) block. **A.** Introduction of a spinal needle (25 G, 3½″) through the coronoid notch, lateral view. **B.** Cross section (caudad to cephalad view) of the spinal needle striking the lateral pterygoid plate, followed by the introduction of the needle tip into the pterygoid fossa.

concentrations of epinephrine mentioned above is injected at the infraorbital foramen, into the pterygoid fossa, and in the region of the great auricular nerve as it emerges from behind the sternomastoid muscle (Fig. 2–8). The technique anesthetizes the mandibular branch of the trigeminal (V) nerve, the maxillary branch of the trigeminal nerve (V), and the great auricular nerve, using a volume of anesthetic of 4 mL, 4 mL, and 8 mL, respectively.

The pterygoid fossa is approached via the condyloid notch. A spinal needle (25 G, 3½″) is introduced through the condyloid notch (Fig. 2–9A) perpendicular to the skin of the area (Fig. 2–9B). The needle passes through the condyloid notch and strikes the lateral surface of the lateral pterygoid plate. By withdrawing the needle slightly and inserting the point in a new site posteriorly (moving the butt of the needle anteriorly) in the horizontal plane ("walking" the needle tip posteriorly), the posterior edge of the lateral pterygoid plate is located (see Fig. 2–9B). The needle is introduced a short distance, to be certain it has passed the lateral pterygoid plate. The pterygoid fossa has a plethora of veins and therefore, prior to injection of the anesthetic solution, aspiration should be done to be certain the needle has not entered a vein. If blood is aspirated, the needle can be withdrawn slightly, and a new site tested. Rarely, it is necessary to withdraw the needle and repeat the introduction at a new site in the condyloid notch.

References

1. Kaye, B.L.: The extended neck lift: The "bottom line." Plast. Reconstr. Surg. 1980; 65:429–435.
2. Skoog, T.: Plastic Surgery—New Methods. Philadelphia, W.B. Saunders, 1974, pp. 309–310, 312.

THREE

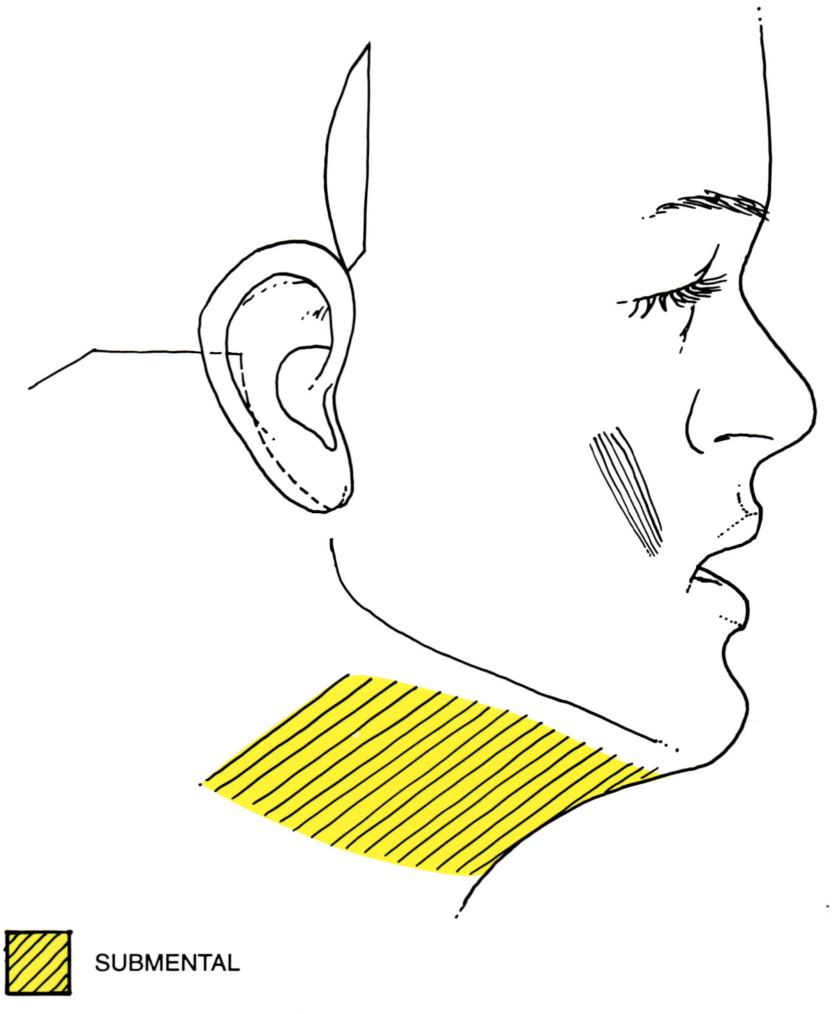

depth of the incision extends to the platysma muscle. Prior to administering the general anesthesia and with the patient in an upright position, the subcutaneous fat deformities (submental fat pad, jowls or midline fat fold) or the platysma muscle folds of the submental region and cervicomental angle of the neck are outlined with the marking solution. Two single skin hooks (sharp), or a double skin hook (sharp)* are placed on the mentum wound edge (Fig. 3–2), and the mandible (and head) hyperextended. After sufficient subdermal undermining of the caudad edge of the submental incision a fiberoptic lighted retractor**,*** is inserted; the blade in the caudad direction (or a fiberoptic headlight is used). This incision provides access to the fat deformities of the jaw line and the neck, and the platysma muscle.

As there is an extensive amount of work to be done through the small submental incision, good lighting is necessary. In the process of developing experience in the restoration of the platysma muscle and cervicomental angle, it may be best to employ both a retractor and a headlight with a fiberoptic light source. Both the lighted retractor and the headlight have their advantages and disadvantages. With the lighted retractor the beam of light is placed directly on the area undergoing dissection (jowl area, anterior cervical preplatysma muscle plane or any area desired). The headlight beam has some restriction in the submental/cervicomental region because of the small incision's aperture, but as a matter of personal preference may be more comfortable for the operator. Certainly in other areas of the rhytidectomy (the cheek, the posterior cervical region and the elevation of the SMAS) it is a

---

*V. Mueller, Baxter Healthcare Corp., Operating Room Division, McGaw Park, IL 60085.
**Rees retractor with fiberoptic, 5¾″ blade, serrated tip, Walter Lorenz Surgical Instruments, Inc., Jacksonville, FL 32218.
***BFW, Wehmerlite IV-A with Maxillume 150-1 light source, BFW, Lexington, KY 40503.

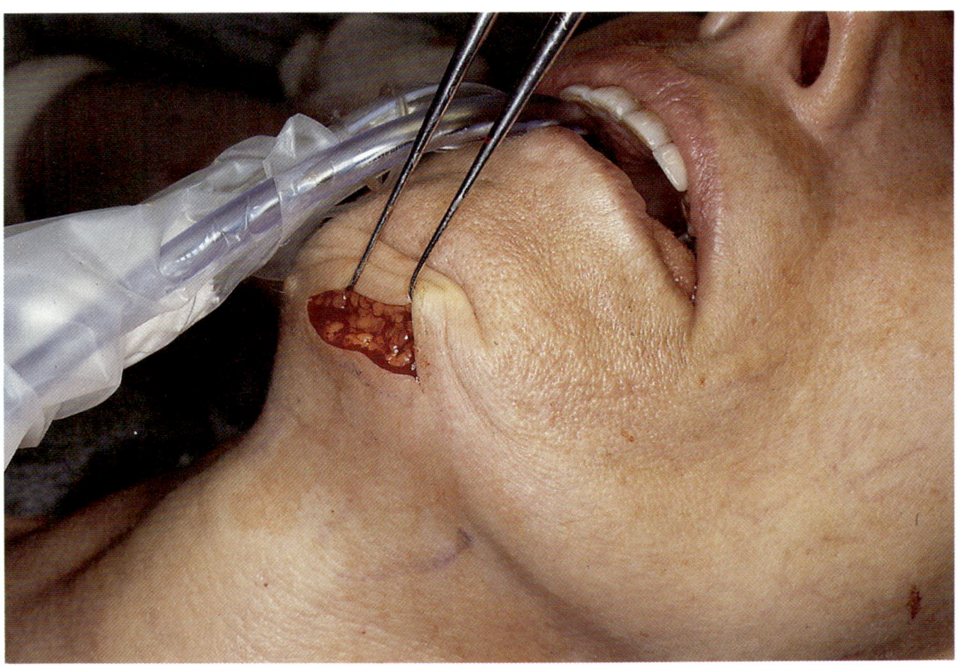

Figure 3–2. The submental incision.

matter of personal preference. Experience using both simultaneously and alternating between the two will determine in time which the operator finds most successful and efficient.

Prior to proceeding further, and because of the restriction imposed by the small incision, the management of electrocoagulation of bleeders should be noted. Unipolar or bipolar electrocoagulation is employed. Because of the proximity of the branches of the facial nerve, bipolar electrocoagulation is utilized at the time of the elevation of the SMAS, and it can be used throughout the procedure. In the submentum/anterior cervical region insulated bipolar bayonet thumb forceps* work well and do not interfere with visibility. In less restricted areas (cheek and posterior cervical area) a bipolar Adson forceps** may be preferred. A power unit*** which incorporates unipolar or bipolar current is useful should the electrocutting current be desired for transecting the anterior border of the platysma muscle or dissecting in the depth of the submental region.

The Mandibular (Jowl) Fat Pad

As aging progresses, the descent of the mandibular fat pad overrides the lower border of the mandible, breaking the smooth contour of the jawline present in the younger person. When the interruption of the jawline is early, or minimal, an extensive SMAS procedure will eliminate the defect entirely. When the patient is older or there are increased amounts of fat in the neck and the mandibular fat pad is large, an extended SMAS procedure will not guarantee a completely smooth jawline. Some reduction of the fat in the area can improve the jaw contour. In this situation a portion (Fig. 3–3) of the fat pad below the lower border of the mandible can be removed under direct vision. The superior portion of the fat pad will be elevated by the SMAS procedure. Allowance should be made for the amount of SMAS elevation expected to ensure that the area of fat removal remains below the inferior border of the mandible.

Submental and Cervical Lipectomy

Fat in the neck (Table 3–2) may present as a submental fat pad, a submental/midline wattle, or a fold of skin and fat extruding from the mentum crease to just above the sternoclavicular joints or to varying levels in the midline of the neck. At the extreme, a "heavy" fatty neck dropping from the lower border of the mandible obscures the usual contours of the underlying anatomy of the neck—the lower border of the mandible and a defined and pleasing cervicomental angle. Last, the fat of the face and neck may be of moderate uniform thickness and quite firm, and in the submental region may present as a firm, round redundant bulge.

---

*Rhoton Bayonet Bipolar, 7⅛ with 1.5–2.0 mm tips. V. Muellar, Baxter Healthcare Corp., Operating Room Division, McGaw Park, IL 60085.

**Adson bipolar thumb forceps, straight, 4¾. Codman & Shurtleff, Inc., Randolph, MA 02368.

***Aspen Labs, a subsidiary of Zimmer, Englewood, CO 80155.

Figure 3–3. Reduction of the "jowl" fat. **A.** Jaw contour deformity ("jowl"). **B.** Partial excision of "jowl" fat.

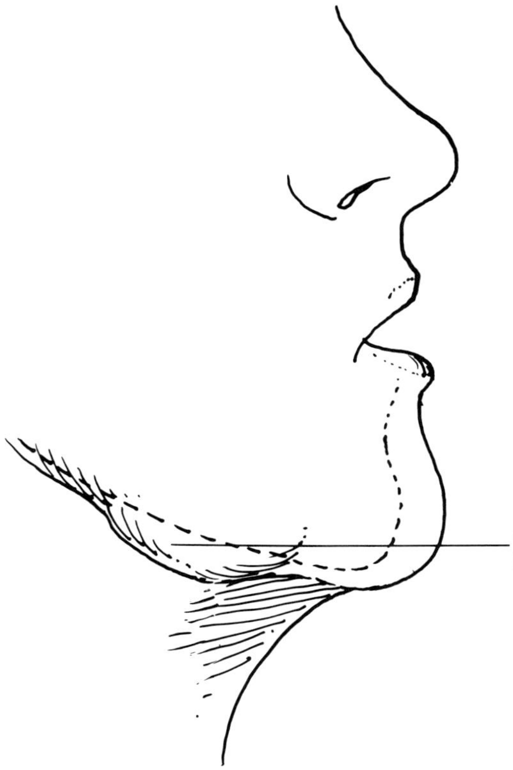

A

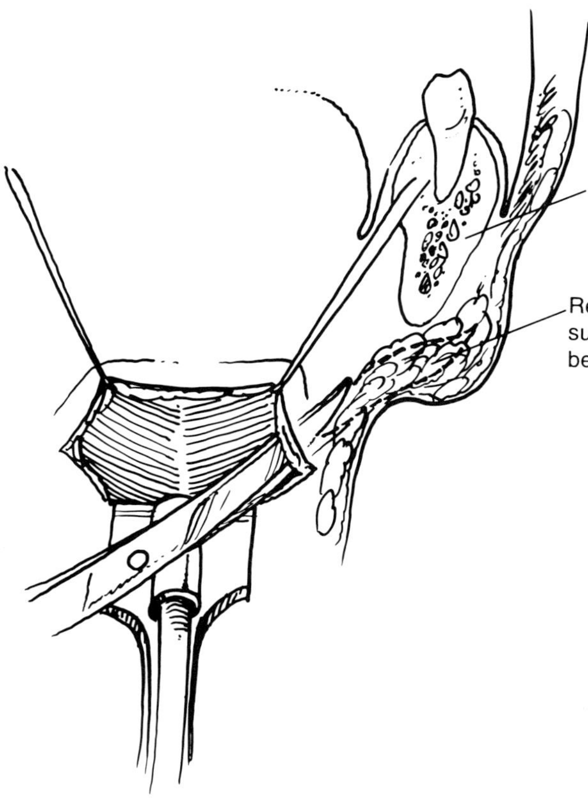

B

Table 3–2. Fatty Deformities of the Submental Region

1. Submental fat pad (small-large)
2. Midline skin and fat fold (ranging from the submentum crease to the midneck crease or to the sternoclavicular area)
3. "Heavy" fatty neck (obscuring the lower border of the mandible and the neck anatomy to the clavicles)
4. Firm submental/cervical fat, moderately thick

The removal of fat in the submental region and neck should be limited, except in extremely fat necks, to the submental fat pad and laterally in the submandibular area approximately 1.5 cm below the mandibular border. After lipectomy, the thickness of the remaining submental fat should be the same as that of the adjacent subcutaneous fat layer of the neck.

In the patient with minimal or slightly increased neck fat, the fat of the neck can be removed by subdermal elevation of the skin over the area and any excess fat removed from the platysma muscle by sharp dissection (or suction lipectomy). With this approach it is difficult to determine the thickness of the fat or the amount to remove; therefore, again it is better to have more than less, or perhaps remove none as upon redraping, a minimal subcutaneous fat layer will appear thinner.

In the fatty, "heavy" neck, and even in the neck with slightly increased amounts of fat, the tendency is to remove too much fat either in the submental or in the anterior cervical, submandibular areas. This, in the extreme, can create a skeletonized appearance and the skin can adhere to the platysma muscle, which upon animation creates a very distracting appearance in the skin "flow" of the neck or over the jawline. Also, overzealous removal may produce irregularities and/or depressions.

A minimal submental fat pad is removed easily by liposuction (Fig. 3–4). A small suction cannula (1.5 mm single lumen, stainless steel) is inserted through the submental incision and into the submental fat pad, and suction is applied while the cannula is directed in a fan pattern in the area of the pad. After 10 to 15 strokes, the cannula is moved approximately 3 to 5 mm to a new point of entry on the incision and the same routine performed. This is continued across the wound until the estimated amount of fat is removed. This technique provides a crisscross, or overlapping suction removal of the fat pad.

Thicker submental fat pads do not always have clearly defined borders and more uniform results can be achieved by a direct-vision excision. After the subcutaneous fat is elevated from the platysma muscle, exposing the anterior borders of the platysma muscle, the plane separating the subdermal fat from the submental fat pad is entered. The skin over the submental region is elevated at the subdermal plane with blunt and sharp dissection (Fig. 3–5).*,** The submental fat pad is removed and the lateral borders of the submental fat

*Wood-Smith-Casson Pow'r Edge, Tungsten Carbide scissors, 6¾" (Mayo-type). Walter Lorenz Surgical Instruments, Inc., Jacksonville, FL 33218.

**Brown-Adson thumb forceps, 4¾". V. Mueller, Baxter Healthcare Corp., Operating Room Division, McGaw Park, IL 60085.

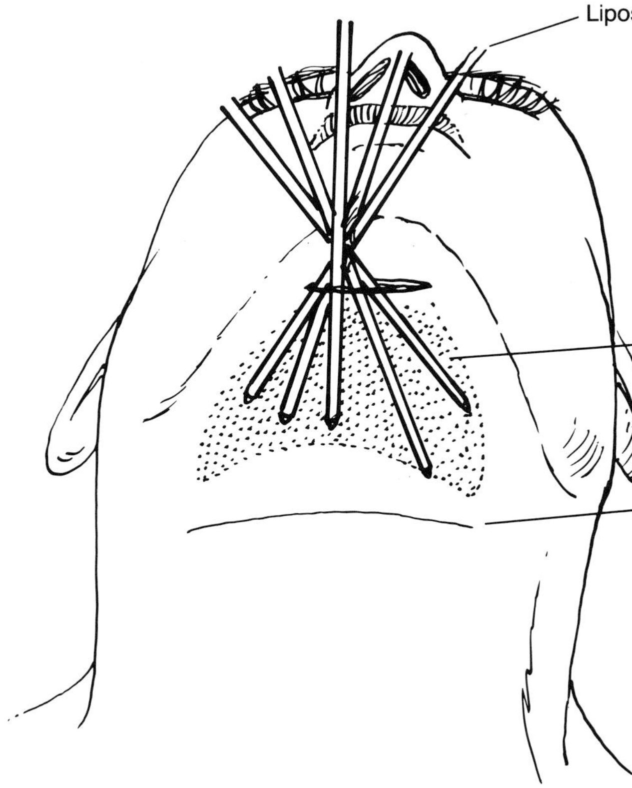

Figure 3–4. Submental lipectomy, suction assisted.

pad pocket feathered. If the subcutaneous fat of the cervical and anterior regions of the neck is thick, this thickness must be maintained in the submental region or the submental area will be depressed. If preferred, the subdermal elevation of the skin can be done first and then the subcutaneous fat elevated from the platysma muscle.

After the removal of submental fat by suction or direct vision, and when little, if any fat, is to be removed from the neck, a suction cannula can be utilized as a dissecting instrument in the anterior region of the neck. Longer and larger (2.4 mm, Mercedes-type tip, stainless steel) cannulas may be fanned out in the subcutaneous tissue of the neck to be elevated, utilizing only a few strokes in each tunnel. The skin now can be easily elevated with the scissors and there seems to be less bleeding than when accomplished by sharp dissection. If a large amount of fat is to be removed, this technique should not be used, as the contusion of the tissues makes it difficult to determine the thickness of the remaining subcutaneous fat and therefore, it is difficult to estimate the amount of fat to remove.

The midline fatty skin fold of the neck (see Table 3–2, item 2) extending caudad from the submentum crease to various levels on the anterior surface of the neck is outlined preoperatively with the patient in the upright position. Lateral to the midline fat and skin fold, the subcutaneous fat layer usually will be of normal thickness. If it is slightly thicker, it should be considered, and probably is, the "normal" thickness for the body type of the patient. The thickness of this layer is the "target" thickness for the skin and subcutaneous fat of the midline of the neck.

Through the submental incision, the skin and subcutaneous fat of the midline wattle and adjacent "normal" skin and subcutaneous fat are elevated from the underlying platysma muscle. Parenthetically, in the patient with a large fatty wattle, the platysma muscle more often than not is thin and does not present as a platysma muscle fold, but is attenuated and embedded in the fat. The elevated skin–subcutaneous fat flap is trimmed of fat by sharp dissection of the deep surface until its thickness approximates the adjacent "normal" subcutaneous fat layer. The thickness is gauged by bimanual palpation.

When the submental area is approached from the posterior incisions about the ear, the subdermal dissection of the postauricular flap is converted to the subcutaneous fat–platysma muscle plane at the anterior border of the sternomastoid muscle. The chapter logo illustrates the area of the skin–subcutaneous fat flap elevation at the preplatysma muscle level in the neck (yellow). At closure, this permits complete redraping of the released skin and subcutaneous fat of a uniform thickness.

The fatty neck obscuring the lower border of the mandible and the anatomical landmarks of the neck (the "heavy" neck) (see Table 3–2, item 3) is managed in a fashion similar to that for the neck with a midline fat and skin fold. The patient with a "heavy" neck usually presents with a thicker layer of facial subcutaneous fat; therefore, the skin–subcutaneous fat layer of the neck should be proportionate to the subcutaneous fat layer of the face. It is possible to leave a moderate subcutaneous fat layer in the neck and yet the neck still looks too thin relative to the face and head. The goal in this situation is to remove only amounts of fat sufficient to establish a visible mandibular border and a more defined cervicomental angle, and to maintain a uniform layer of subcutaneous fat in the face and neck.

The skin–subcutaneous fat layer is separated from the platysma muscle and the subcutaneous fat layer thinned from the undersurface (deep). This is done with sharp dissection; however, judicious liposuction on the deep surface of the skin–subcutaneous fat flap can be of assistance. The results in the operator's practice will depend on judgment and experience both in evaluating the amount of fat to be removed and in correlating this and the postoperative appearance of the skin–subcutaneous fat layer of the neck. Again, only so much fat is removed as is necessary to meet the "target" thickness present in the face, or an area on the neck considered to be the uniform thickness of the subcutaneous fat for the individual's body type.

When the patient has a moderately thick subcutaneous fat layer that is of uniform thickness over the neck and is firm, and the submental area has a firm, round, bulging redundancy, the thick firm fat can be difficult to reduce in volume without causing postoperative deformities.* If the submental area is defatted, the firm fat laterally is thicker and the submental area is depressed. Also reduced firm fat tends to retain "carved" contours and postoperatively, even with smoothing of the tissues with time, may cause undulating areas and sometimes crater deformities. In these circumstances, to reduce the risk of postoperative defects and to ensure that the thick, firm subcutane-

*The correction of all the fat and platysma muscle deformities of the submental and anterior cervical region of the neck follow the same operative sequence to be described for the management of the subcutaneous fat of the neck which is thick and firm.

ous fat layer will be a thickness consistent with that of the surrounding fat, which has not been reduced in volume, the submental volume of fat can be reduced by creating two quadrilateral flaps of the subcutaneous fat layer that are based laterally.

The skin in the submental region is elevated at the subdermal level (see Fig. 3–5). Next, the subcutaneous fat layer is elevated from the platysma muscle. The dissection is extended as far as possible in a caudad direction (see Fig. 3–5). The subcutaneous fat is incised in the midline from the mentum to the cervicomentum angle. The thick subcutaneous fat layer is incised next, along a line parallel to and approximately 1.5 cm below the inferior border of the mandible and at the level of the cervicomental angle. This produces two quadrilateral fat flaps based laterally. Upon completion of a subplatysma muscle lipectomy, if necessary, and reconstruction of the platysma muscle, the fat flaps are pulled across the midline just as the platysma is and the midline border of the fat flap is trimmed. A substantial amount of fat is removed and the flaps sutured in the midline. These advanced and joined subcutaneous fat flaps reduce the excess submental fat and preserve the "normal" thickness of the subcutaneous fat layer present in the surrounding areas of the neck. The complete intraoperative sequence of the management of the submental region (platysma muscle, thick firm subcutaneous fat, and sub–platysma muscle fat) follows.

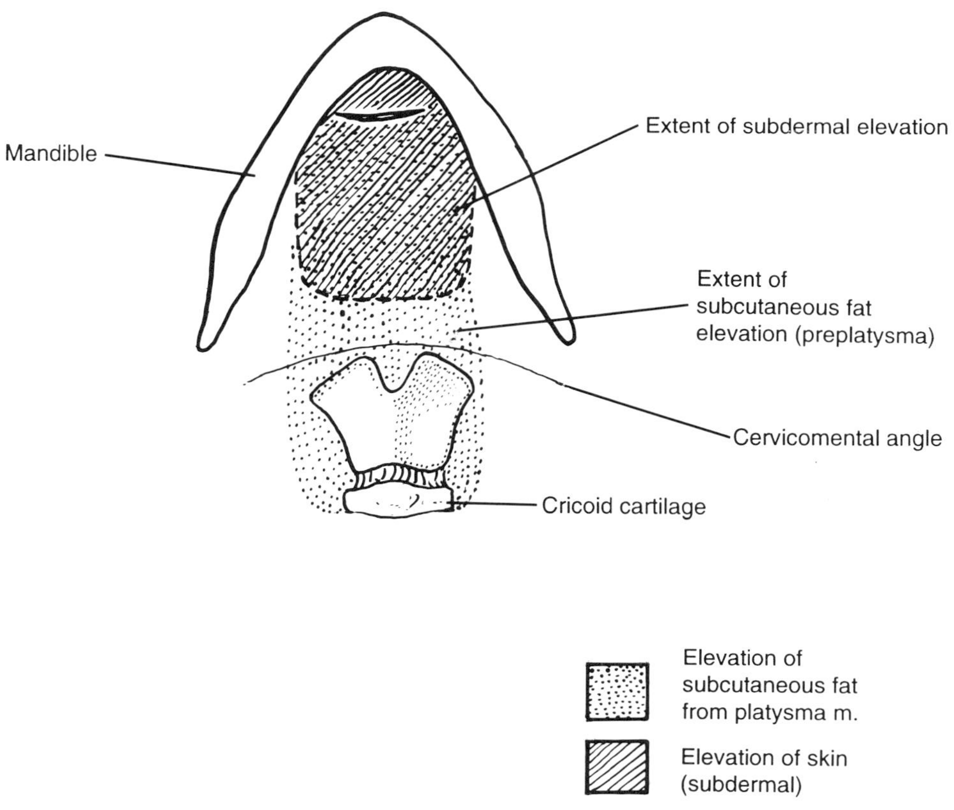

Figure 3–5. The extent of the elevation of the skin/subcutaneous fat flap of the neck and of the subdermal dissection of the submental region.

The Management of the Platysma Muscle and the Subcutaneous and Subplatysma Fat of the Neck: Intraoperative Sequence

Step 1: After subdermal elevation of the skin of the submental region and neck, firm subcutaneous fat of moderate thickness in the neck and an accumulation of relaxed skin and subcutaneous fat in the submental region can be managed by incising the subcutaneous fat in the midline and creating two quadrilateral lateral flaps based laterally (Fig. 3–6).

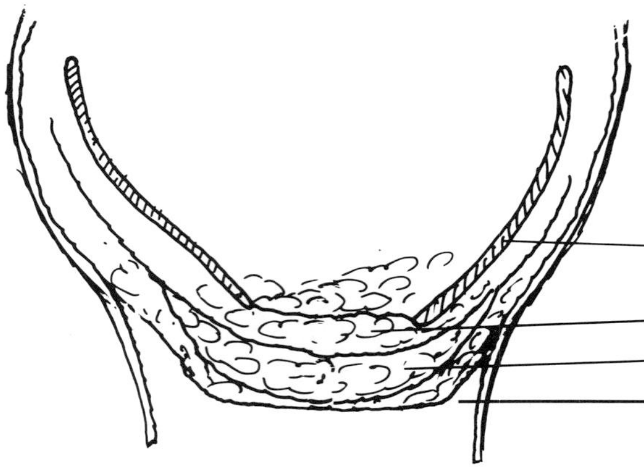

Figure 3–6. The development of bilateral subcutaneous fat flaps (thick, firm fat) of the submental region. **A.** Cross section of (B) and (C). **B.** Proposed incisions (dotted lines) for bilateral submental quadrilateral fat flaps based laterally. **C.** Midline incision of thick, firm fat of the submental region.

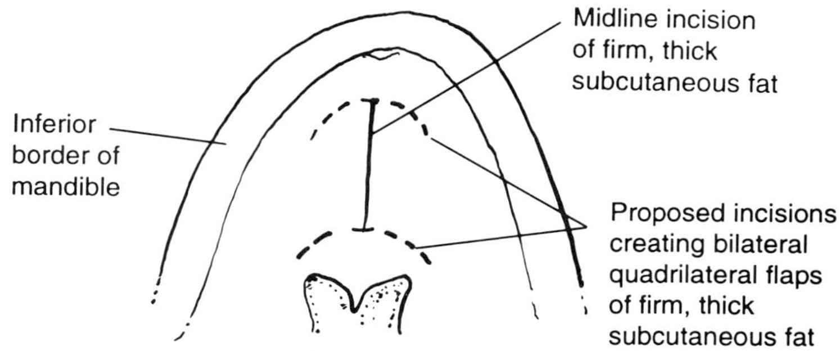

Midline incision of firm, thick subcutaneous fat
Inferior border of mandible
Proposed incisions creating bilateral quadrilateral flaps of firm, thick subcutaneous fat

B

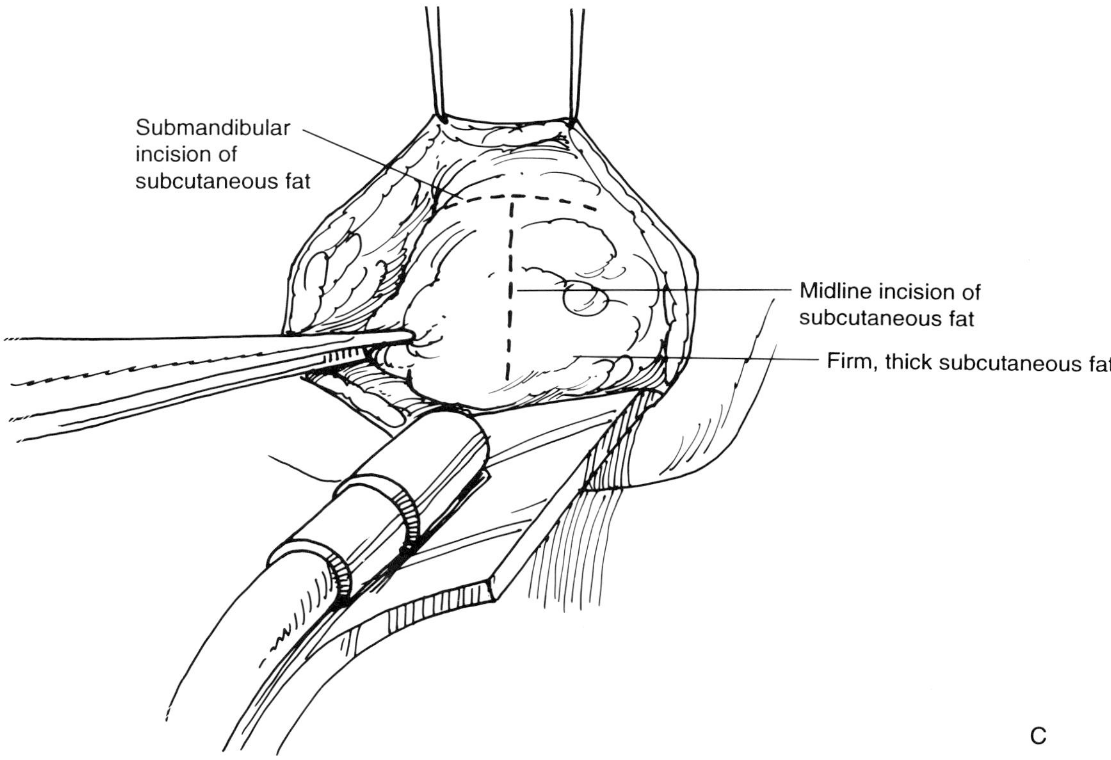

Submandibular incision of subcutaneous fat
Midline incision of subcutaneous fat
Firm, thick subcutaneous fat

C

Step 2: The separated anterior borders of the platysma muscle are identified and elevated from the underlying submuscular fat (Fig. 3–7).*,** Subcutaneous fat has been elevated from the platysma muscle superficially and retracted laterally to expose the musculature. Subplatysma fat is exposed between the anterior borders of the platysma muscle.

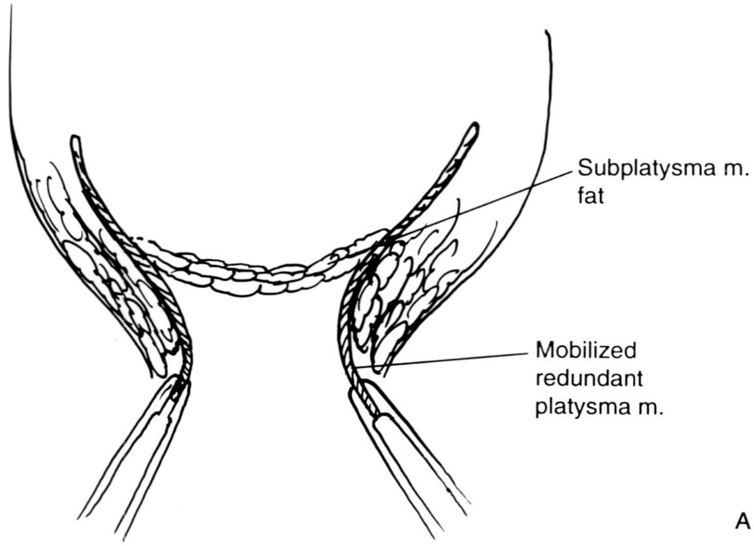

Figure 3–7. Mobilization of the redundant platysma muscle. **A.** Cross section of (B) and (C).

*Kaye Face Lift Scissors, 7″ curved, serrated blades, Snowden-Pencer, Inc., Tucker, GA 30084.
**DeBakey thumb forceps, 7¾″, 2.3 mm tip, Snowden-Pencer, Inc., Tucker, GA 30084.

Figure 3–7 (continued) **B.** Illustration of the intraoperative photograph (C). **C.** Intraoperative photograph.

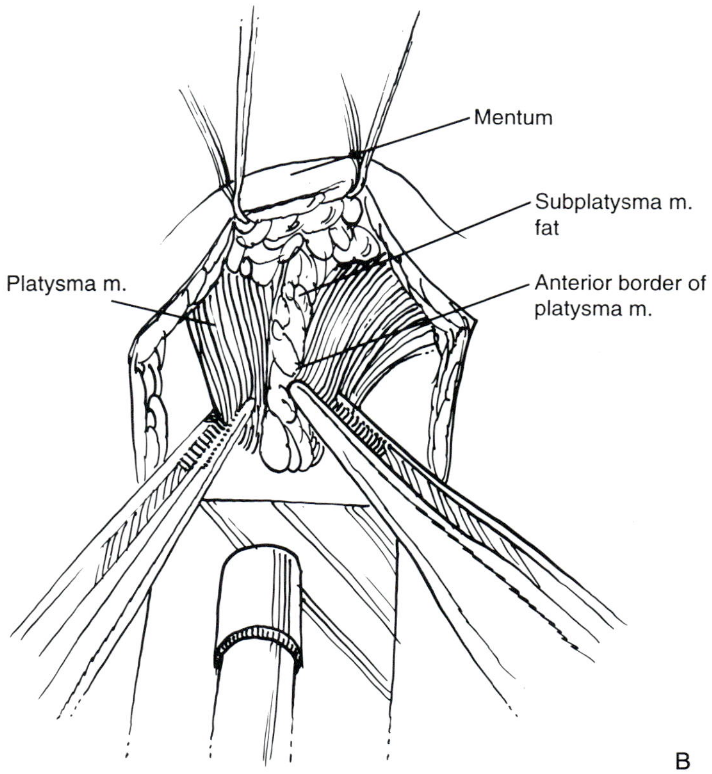

B

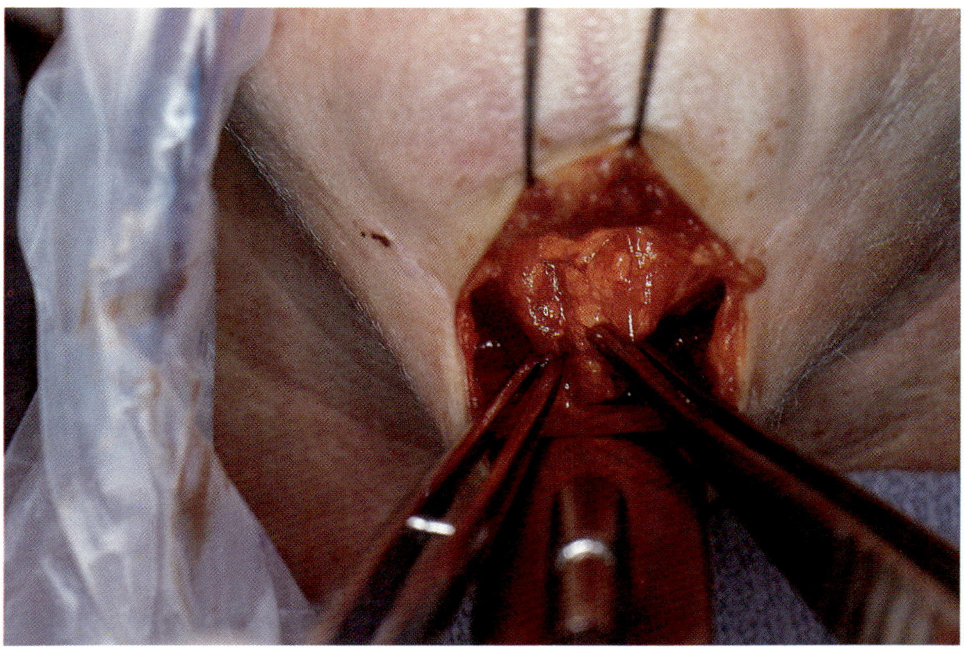

C

Step 3: The elevated platysma muscle is advanced across the midline to estimate the amount of muscle to be excised (Fig. 3–8). The subcutaneous fat layer (freed from the platysma and the skin) is delivered into the wound to show the thickness (approximately 1 cm) and redundancy of the subcutaneous fat layer.

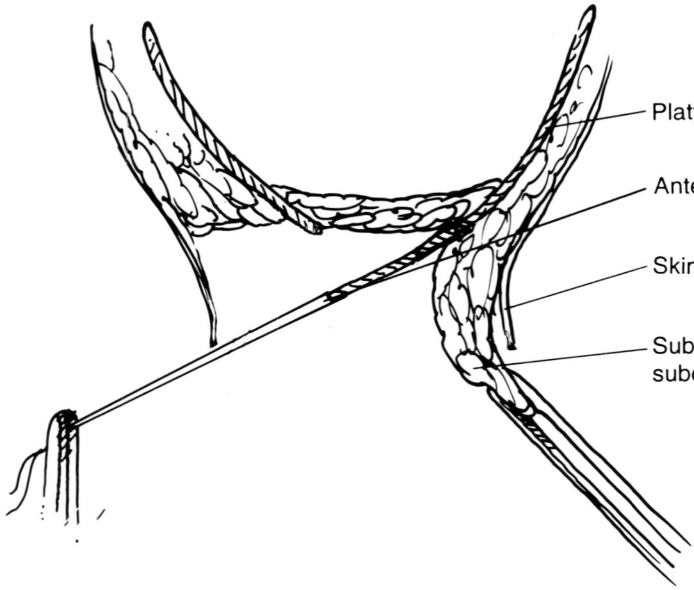

Figure 3–8. Mobilization of the quadrilateral subcutaneous fat flap of the submental region. **A.** Cross section of (B) and (C).

Figure 3–8 (continued) **B.** Illustration of the intraoperative photograph (C). **C.** Intraoperative photograph.

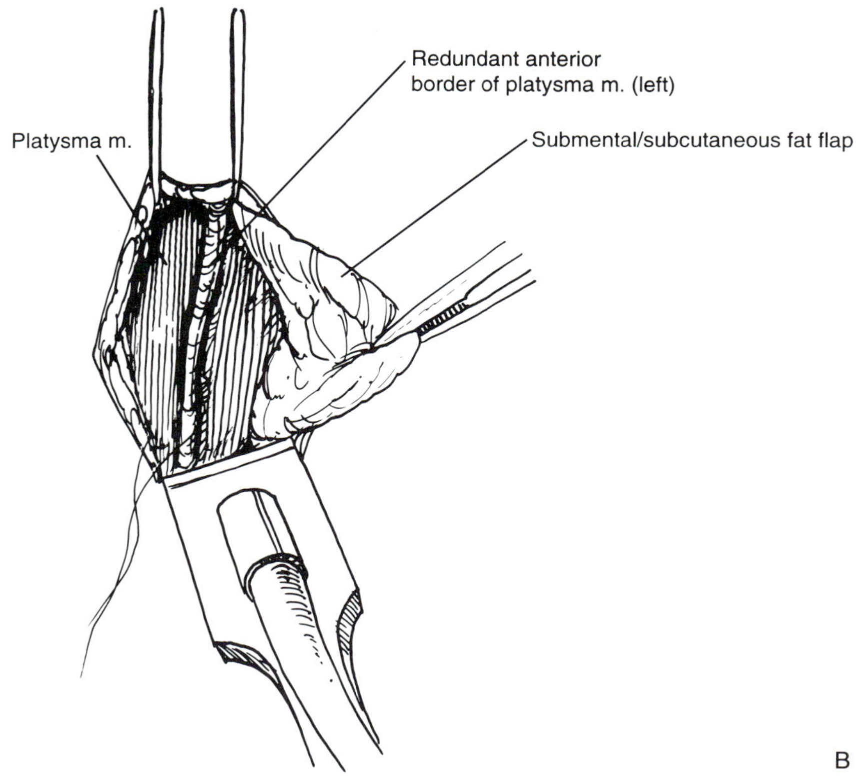

B

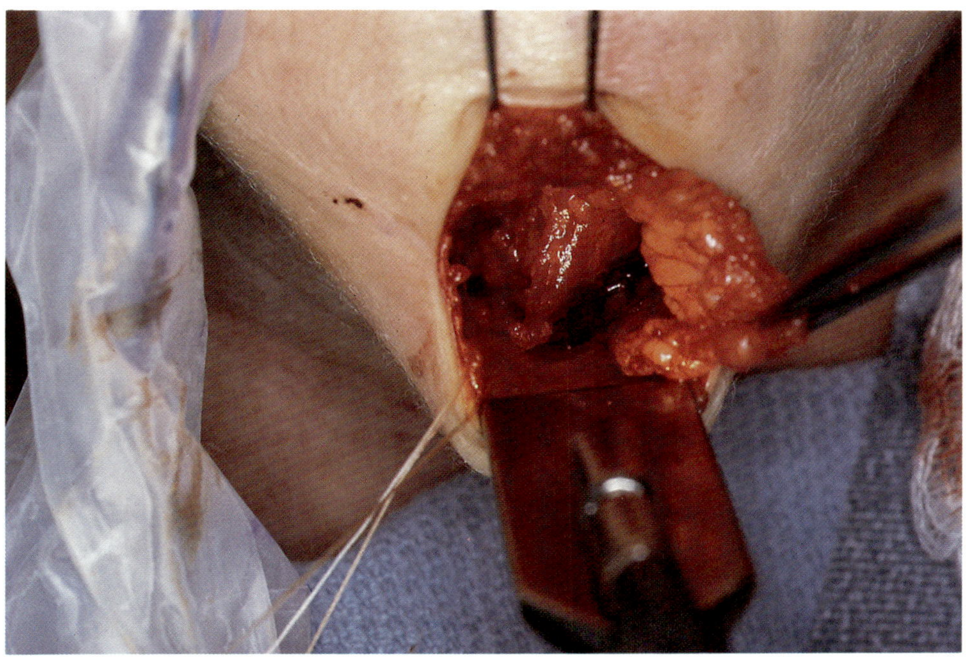

C

Step 4: The advanced anterior border of the platysma muscle is resected from the mentum to the level of the midneck crease (Fig. 3–9). At the level of the cervicomental crease, the anterior edge of the platysma is transected laterally 2.5 to 3.0 cm (see Fig. 3–12). A wedge of muscle is excised from the superior aspect of the transected platysma muscle. This lengthens the anterior border of the platysma, permitting the muscle to meet the curvature of the underlying anatomy of the cervicomental angle, and reduces the tension on the approximation of the platysma edges from the mentum to the cervicomental angle level.

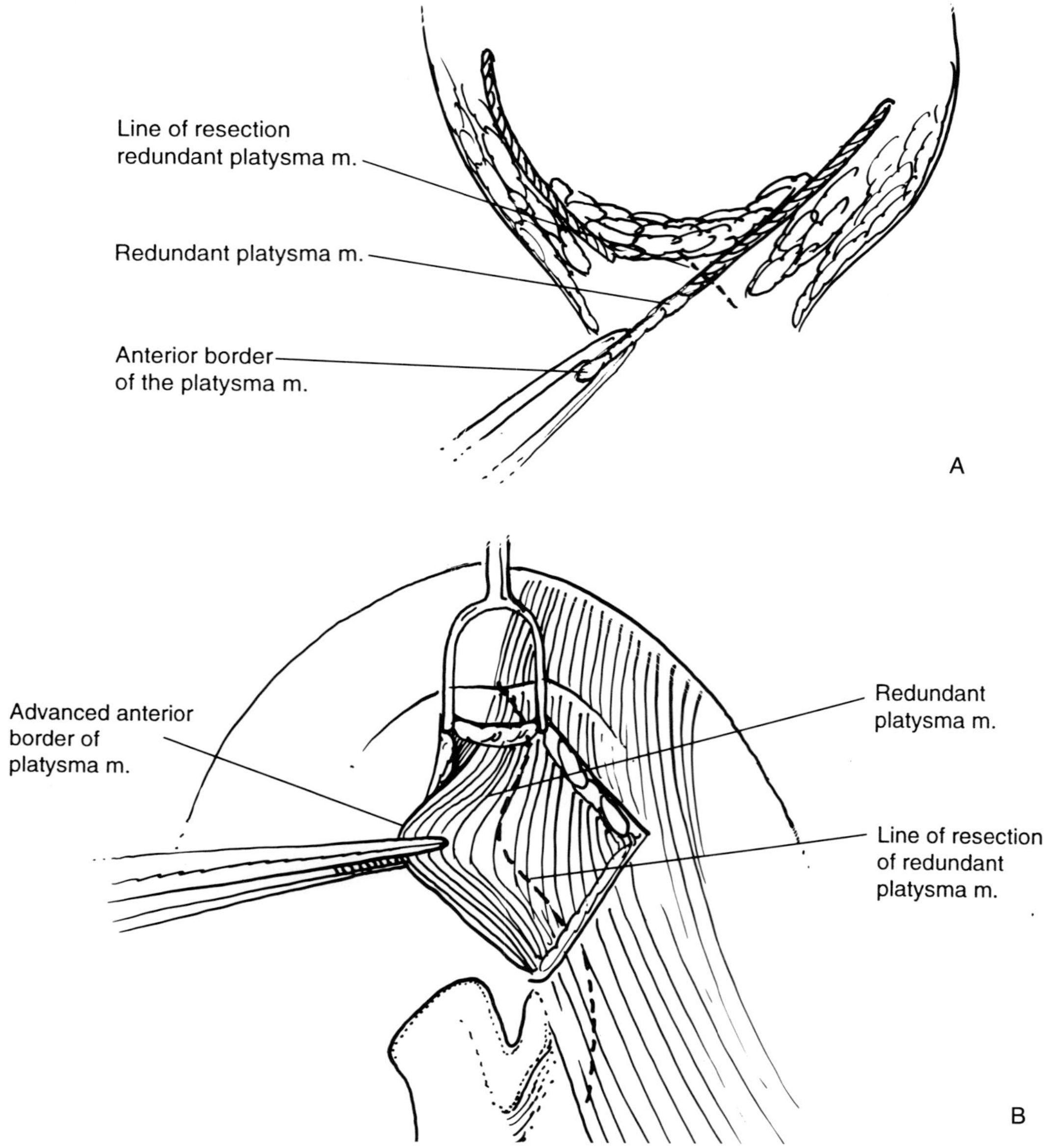

Figure 3–9. Resection of the redundant anterior border of the platysma muscle. **A.** Cross section of (B), (C) and (D). **B.** Dotted line indicates the extent of platysma resection.

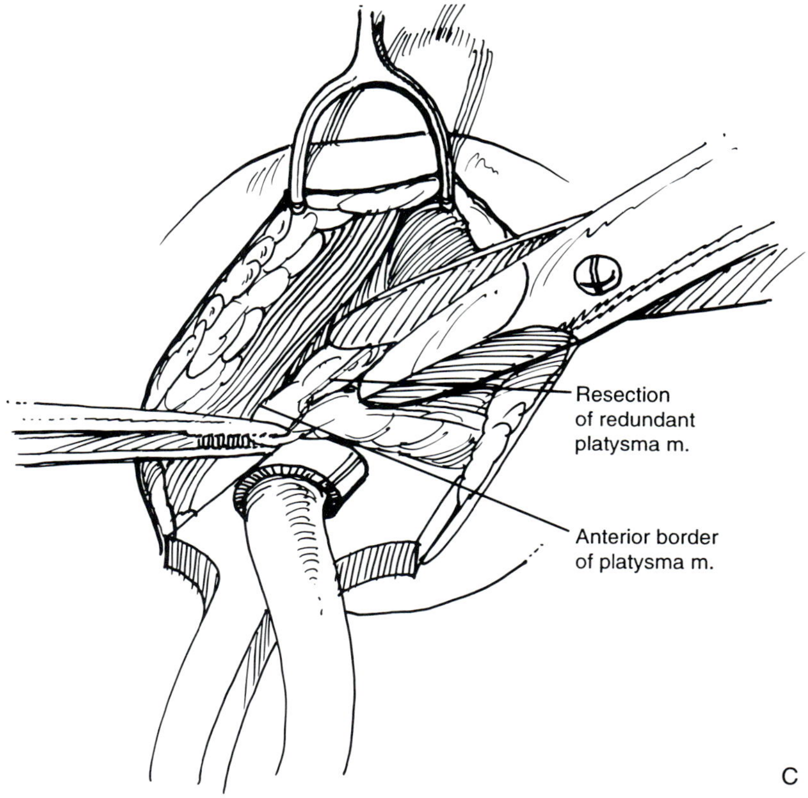

C

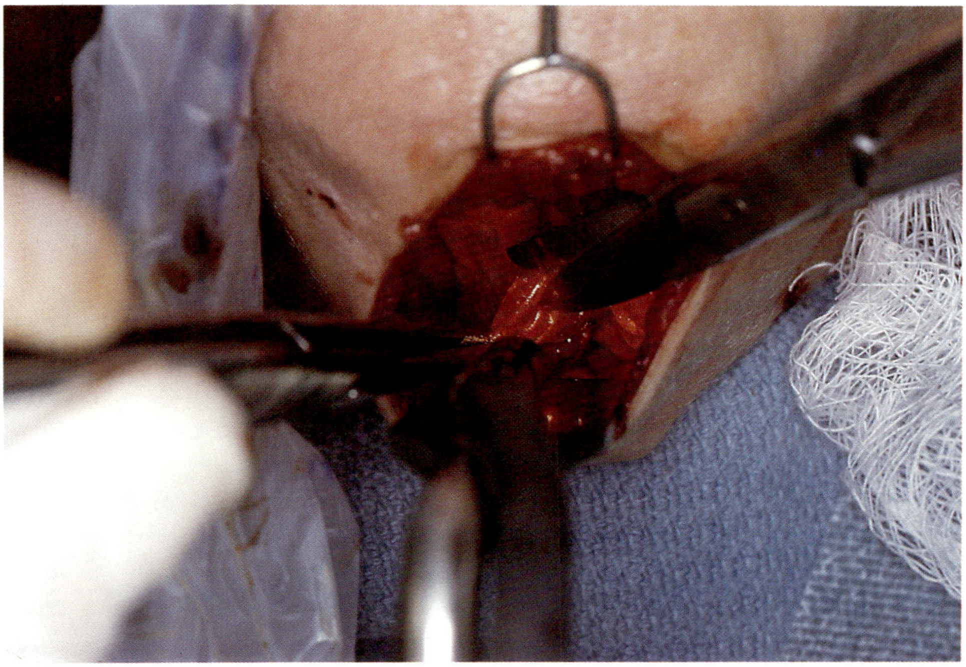

D

Figure 3–9 (continued) **C.** Illustration of the intraoperative photograph (D). **D.** Intraoperative photograph.

Step 5: Subplatysma lipectomy may be indicated to provide the desired submental contour (Fig. 3–10). To avoid a depressed submental region, the subplatysma fat removal is usually limited to no more than approximately one-half of the thickness, or to an appropriate thickness depending on the overall thickness of the individual's subcutaneous fat layers in the neck. This prevents depression and adhesion of the submental region, which upon swallowing accentuates the defect. Also, with the passage of time, relaxation of the tissues lateral to the submental region makes any depression of the region appear relatively more severe than it actually appears early postoperatively.

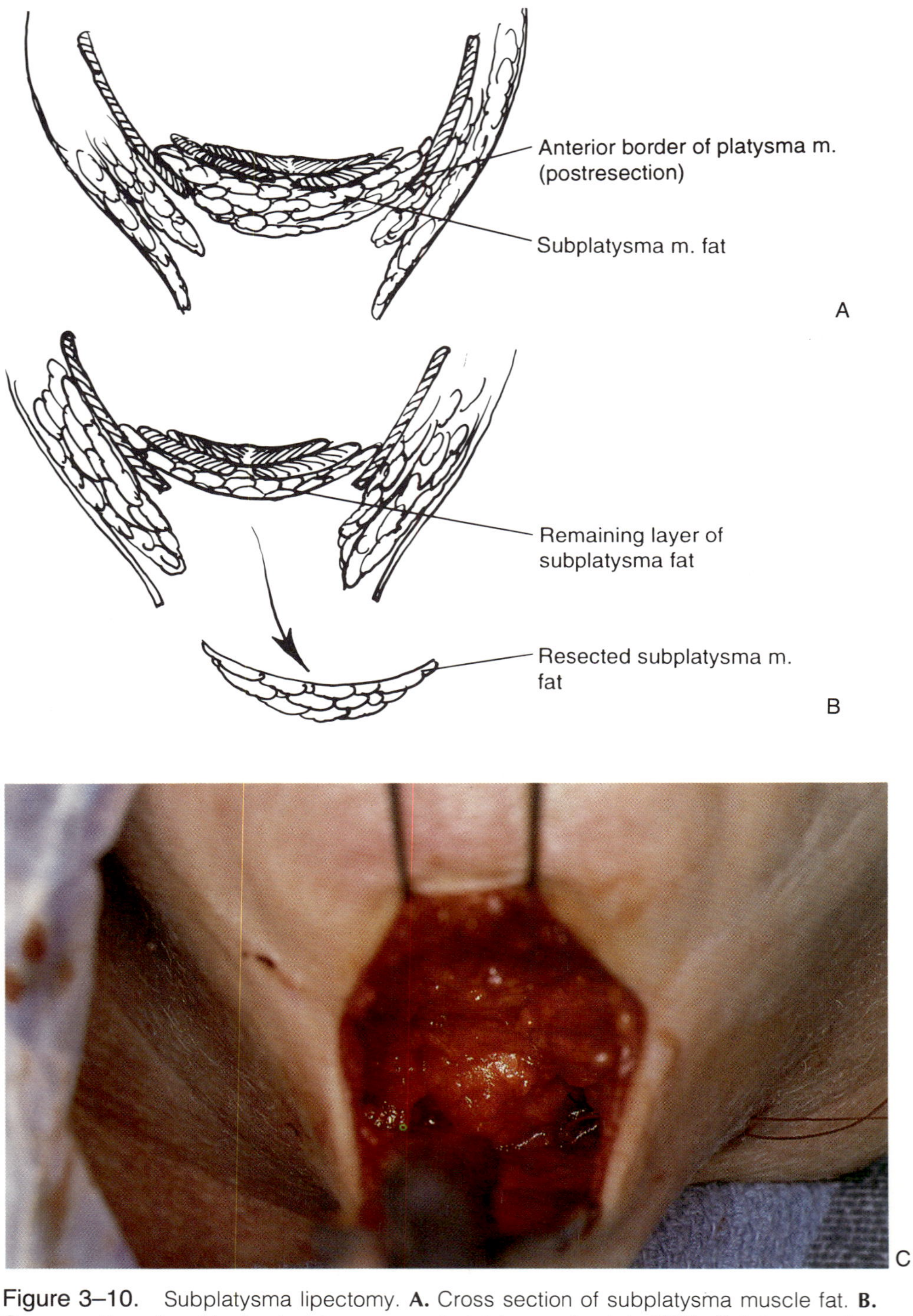

Figure 3–10. Subplatysma lipectomy. **A.** Cross section of subplatysma muscle fat. **B.** Cross section of residual subplatysma muscle fat (approximately 50%). **C.** Intraoperative photograph.

Step 6: The anterior borders of the platysma muscle are closed [4-0 Vicryl sutures (no. 496, Ethicon), interrupted] from the mentum to the cervicomental angle (Fig. 3–11). The inferior border (caudad) of the muscle closure is under moderate tension. If the muscle bowstrings over the deep structures, it can be tacked to the deep fascia. As a result of the myectomy of the anterior border of the platysma muscle and a partial transection with a removal of a wedge of muscle at the level of the cervicomental angle (Fig. 3–12), the tension of the approximation of the platysma muscle above the cervicomental angle places the anterior edge of the platysma below the approximated platysma borders in a superolateral direction, which at times may not be greatly above horizontal. This produces an excellent cervicomental angle, and removes the anterior border of the platysma muscle below the cervicomental angle from the anterior region of the neck. The approximated borders of the platysma muscle extending from the mentum to the cervicomental angle remove the laxity of the muscle from the submental area and along the mandibular border and of the immediate submandibular area. This combination of tightening the platysma muscle above the cervicomental angle and placing anterior borders of the platysma in a more normal anatomical splayed position lateral to the anterior region of the neck results in a very attractive neck that will remain so over many years. The skin cover of the underlying structures below the cervicomental angle appears normal.

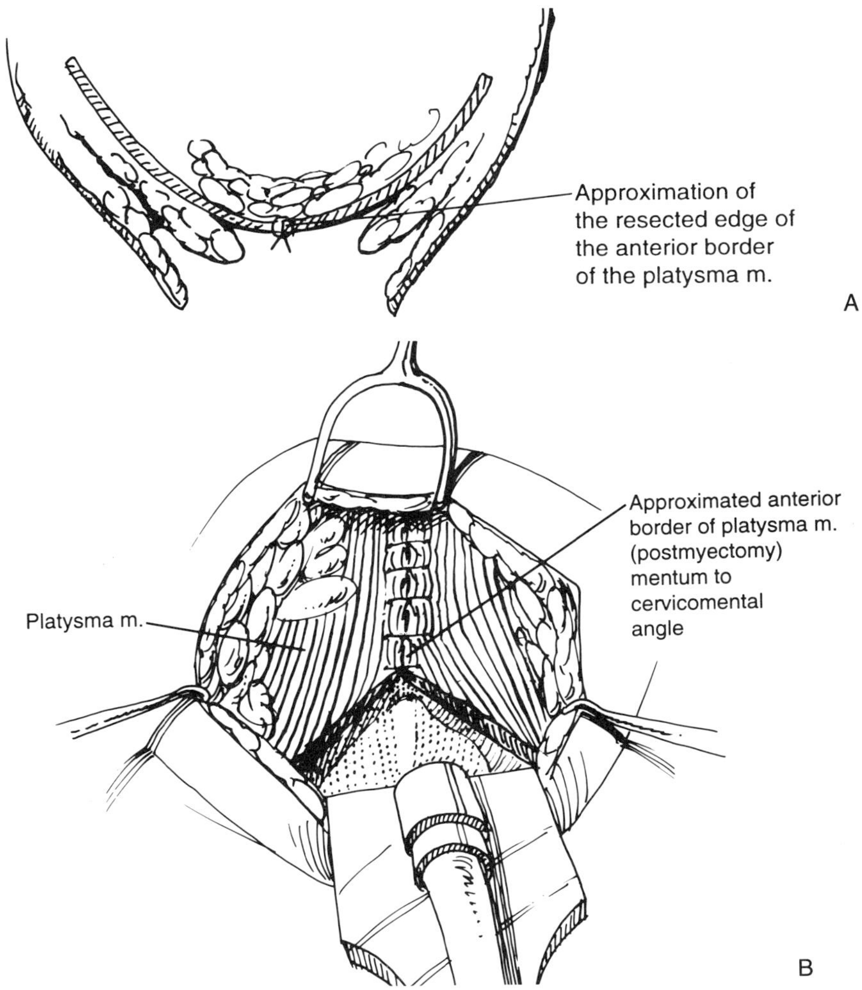

Figure 3–11. Approximation of the resected edge of the anterior border of the platysma muscle. **A.** Cross section of (B) and (C). **B.** Illustration of the intraoperative photograph (C).

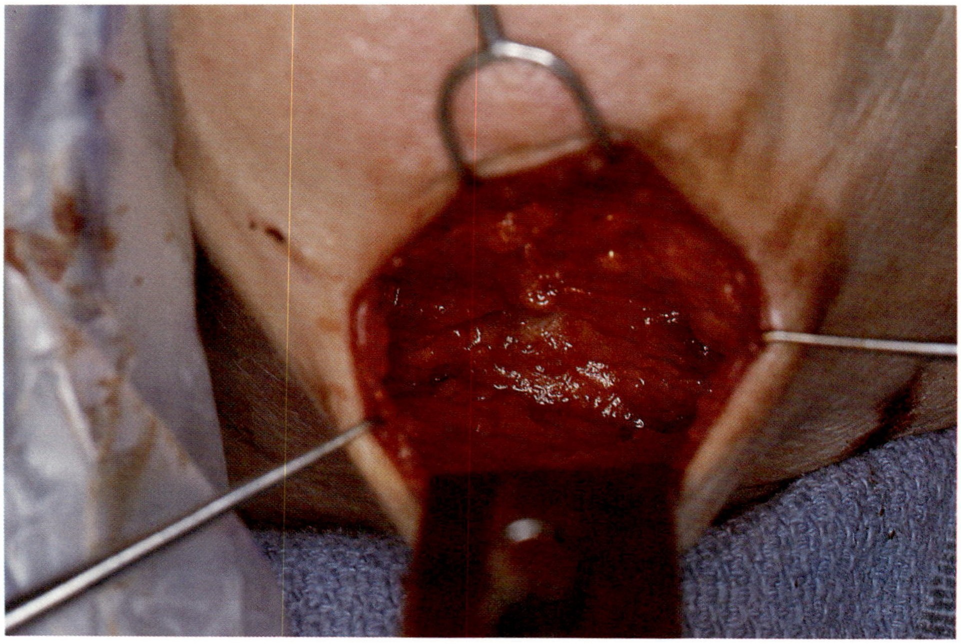

C

Figure 3–11 (continued) **C.** Intraoperative photograph.

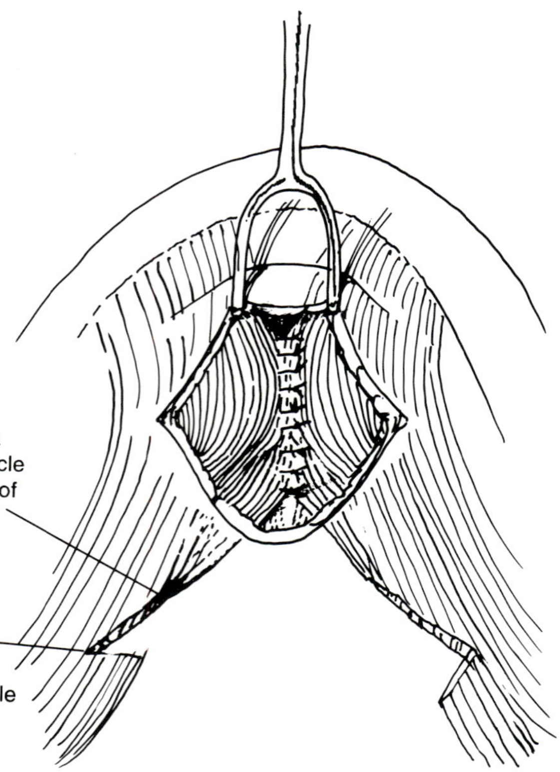

Figure 3–12. Partial transection of the anterior border of the platysma at the level of the cervicomental angle. This may be done in conjunction with the myectomy of the anterior borders of the platysma muscle (Figure 3–9), or after the approximation of the new anterior borders of the platysma muscle above the cervicomental angle.

Step 7: The subcutaneous fat flap created by the subdermal elevation of the skin in the submental region of the neck and the elevation of the thick subcutaneous fat layer from the platysma permits advancement of the bilateral subcutaneous fat flaps across the midline to estimate the amount of excess fat to be excised (Fig. 3–13).

The midline borders of the quadrilateral flaps, based laterally, of thick firm subcutaneous fat are trimmed (Fig. 3–13). This removes the excess fat of the submental region.

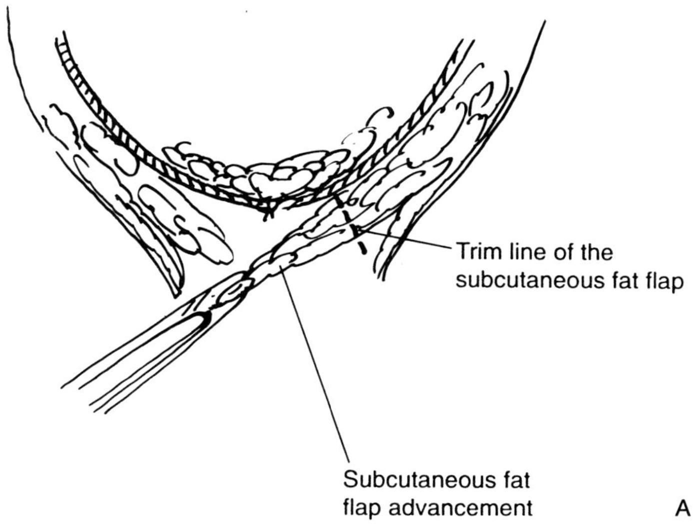

Figure 3–13. Resection of the redundant (advanced) subcutaneous fat flap. **A.** Cross section of (B) and (C).

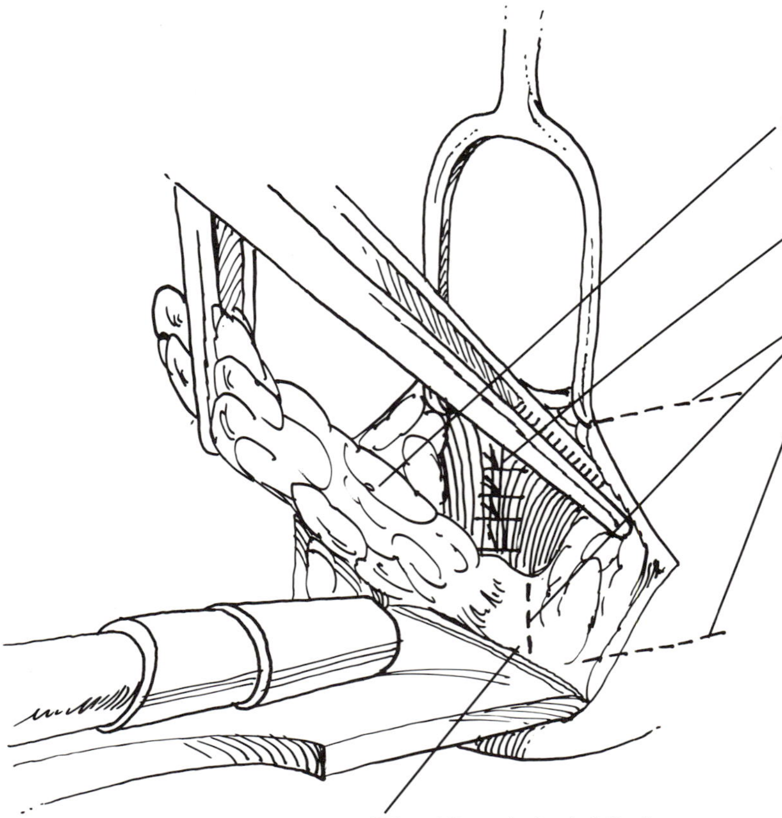

B

Figure 3–13 (continued) **B.** Illustration of the intraoperative photograph (C). **C.** Intraoperative photograph.

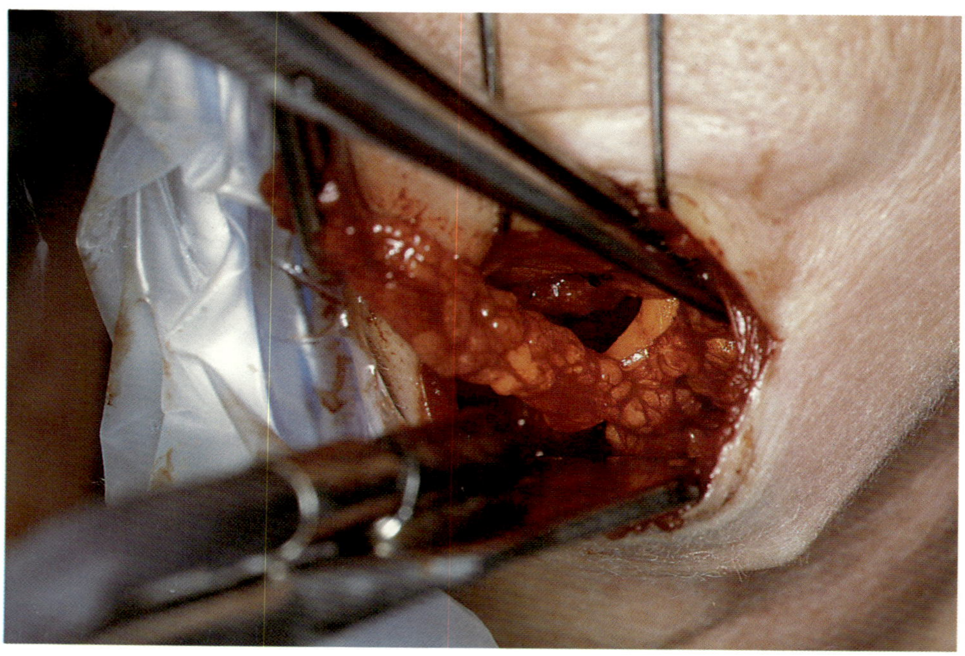

C

Step 8: The subcutaneous fat flap is closed in the midline (Fig. 3–14). With a thicker layer of fat in the submental region, this technique maintains the preoperative thickness of the subcutaneous layer, particularly when the fat consistency is firm, yet sufficient fat is removed to provide a nice neck contour. With this technique there is no guess work as to how thick the layer should be because the redundant fat that was excised is replaced with fat of the same thickness. The reduction in the volume of fat in the midline corrects the round fat protrusion of the submental region.

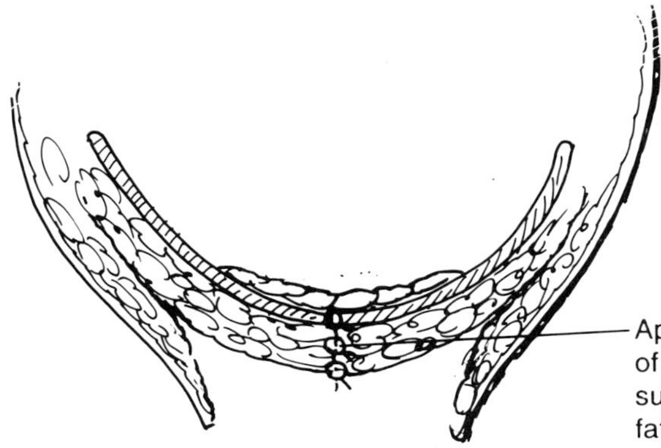

Figure 3–14. Approximation of the advanced subcutaneous fat flaps. **A.** Cross section of (B) and (C).

Figure 3–14 (continued) **B.** Illustration of the intraoperative photograph (C). **C.** Intraoperative photograph.

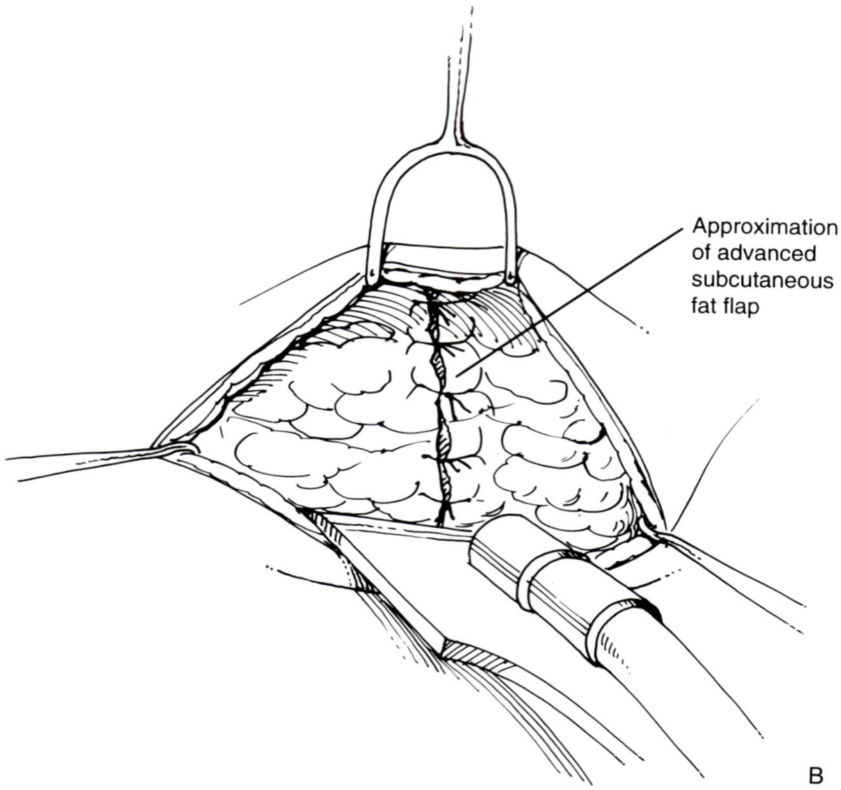

B

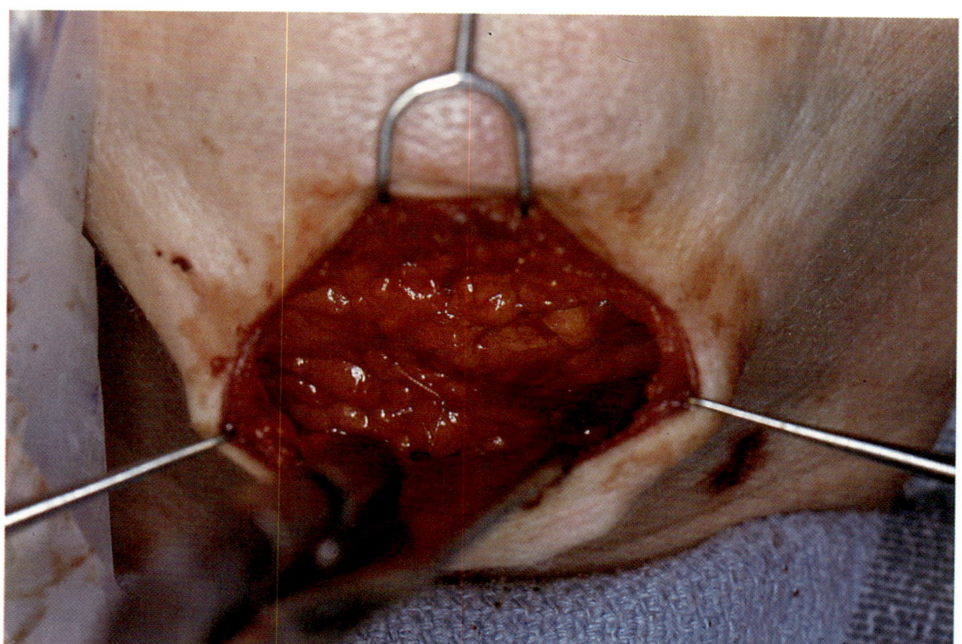

C

Release of the Submental Crease

A fibrous tissue attachment exists between the submental crease and the periosteum of the mandible (Fig. 3–15A). Prior to closure of the submental incision, the attachment is released (Fig. 3–15B, C). (If augmentation of the mentum is planned, the attachment would be released at the time of implantation.) This release provides a better drape of the submental region and diminishes the accent of the crease in the profile view, providing a younger-looking mandible line.

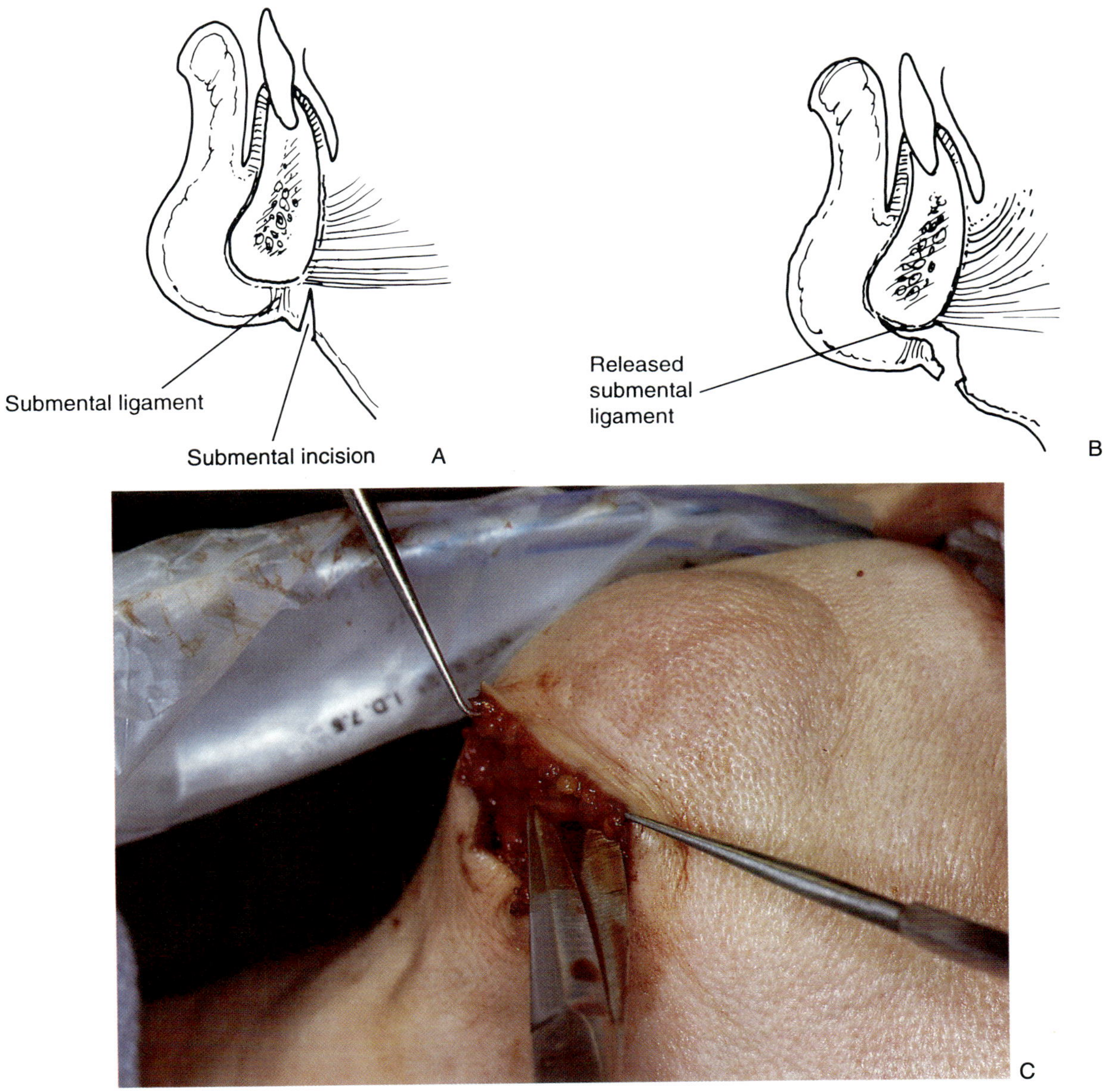

Figure 3–15. The release of the submental crease. **A.** Illustration of the ligamentous attachment of the submental crease to the mandible. **B.** Illustration of the released ligamentous attachment. **C.** Intraoperative photograph of the release of the ligamentous attachment of the submental crease to the mandible.

FOUR

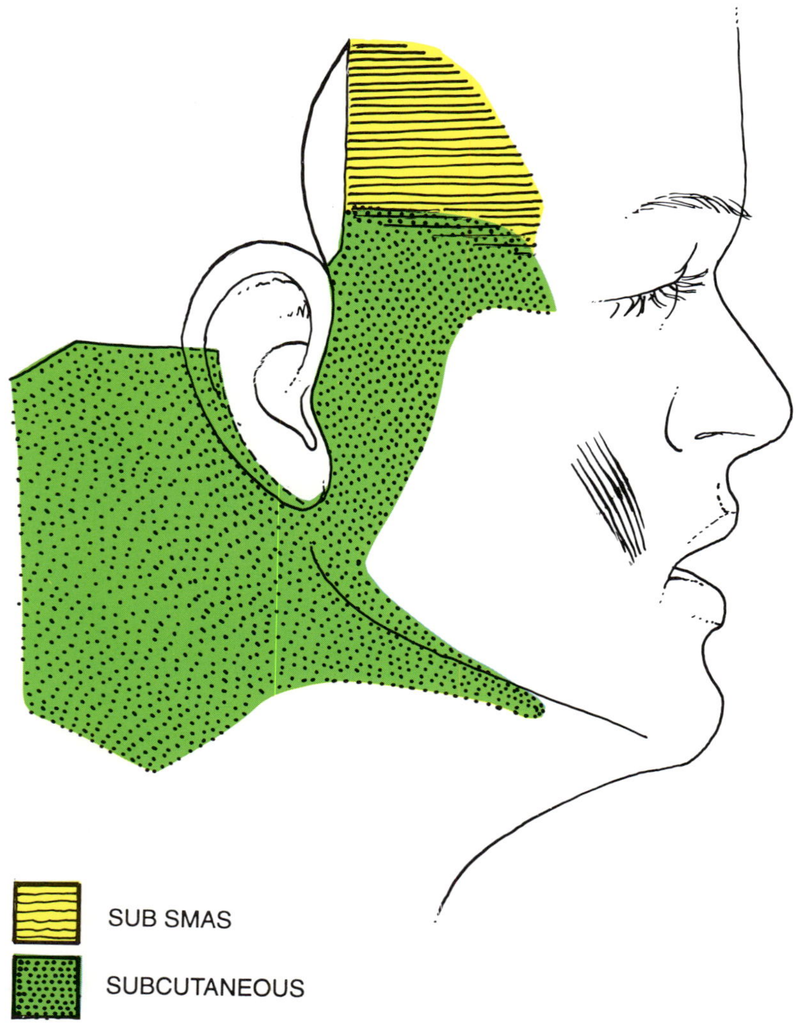

Elevation of the Superficial Temporal Fascia and the Subcutaneous Dissection of the Face and Posterior Cervical Region

Upon completion of the restoration of the submental and neck contours, the procedure is directed to the elevation of the superficial temporal fascia and of the cheek and posterior cervical skin flaps. This chapter describes the techniques involved and the extent of the dissection necessary to provide access to the SMAS and afford a smooth redraping of the skin at wound closure. The neck and the right side of the face are done first and the wounds closed. The left side follows. Table 4–1 details the intraoperative sequence of the rhytidectomy of the face and neck in the temporal, cheek, and posterior cervical areas. Fig. 4–1 indicates the area and the level of the dissection described in this chapter.

Excision of the Redundant (Estimated) Temporal Scalp

The skin incisions are made to the level of the superficial temporal fascia.* The area of the redundant scalp tissue is placed under moderate traction and

*The dissection in Chapter 4 employs the core set of instruments listed in Chapter 3.

Table 4–1. Intraoperative Sequence of the Temporal and the Subcutaneous Areas of the Cheek and the Posterior Cervical Region

1. Temporal, preauricular and postauricular, and occipital incisions
2. Excision of the redundant scalp in the temporal region
3. Penetration and elevation of the superficial temporal fascia
4. Partial subcutaneous dissection of the cheek
5. Skeletonizing of the tragus cartilage in a tragus rim incision
6. Subcutaneous dissection of the postauricular and posterior cervical region
7. Completion of the subcutaneous dissection of the cheek in preparation for the sub-SMAS dissection

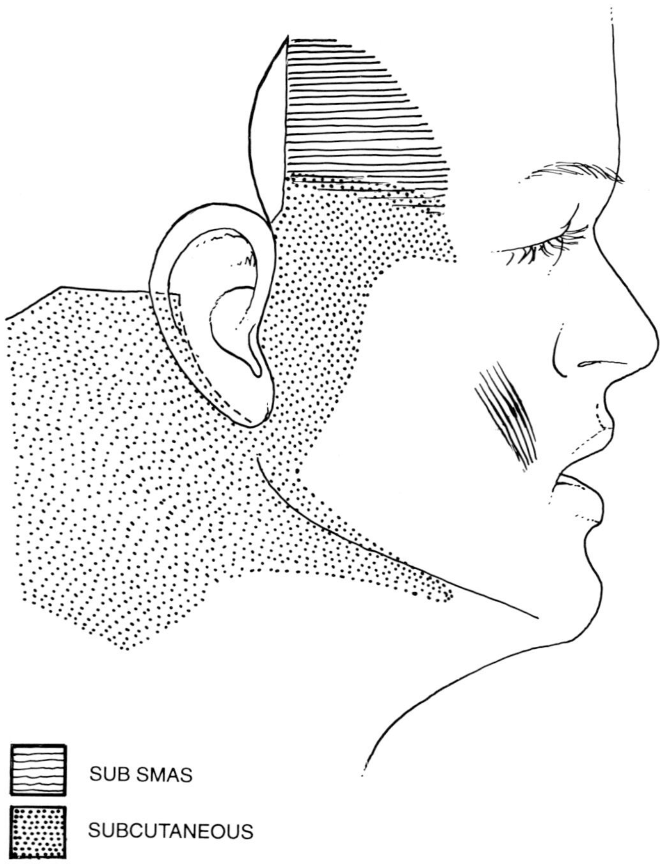

Figure 4–1. The extent of the elevation of the superficial temporal fascia and of the subcutaneous dissection of the cheek and the posterior cervical region.

countertraction by an assistant and is readily peeled off the loose areolar connective tissue overlying the superficial temporal fascia (Fig. 4–2). The superficial temporal artery and vein usually underlie this area of scalp removal. If they are injured, ligation of the vessels may be necessary.

Penetration and Elevation of the Superficial Temporal Fascia

The superficial temporal fascia is usually penetrated in the upper half and along the anterior border of the area of excised redundant scalp (Fig. 4–3A). The plane between the superficial and deep temporal fasciae (Fig. 4–3B) is easily separated from cephalad to caudad. The caudad extent of the opening of the superficial temporal fascia (temporoparietal) is the zygoma (junction of the helix rim of the ear with the skull). Opening the superficial temporal fascia transects the frontal terminal branch of the superficial temporal artery and vein. If electrocautery does not control the bleeding, it may be necessary to ligate the vessels. The loose areolar tissue between the superficial (temporoparietal) fascia and the deep temporal fascia is separated (Fig. 4–4) by penetration and spreading of the scissor blades. The fascia can be elevated further by blunt finger dissection (Fig. 4–5). If there is considerable laxity of the tissues about the orbital and temporal regions, the sub–superficial temporal fascia elevation is extended to the orbital rim. With extensive elevation of the area, the orbicularis oculi is partially elevated. (See Chapter 6, Placement of the Temporal Suture.)

Tragal Rim Incision Technique

Following the excision of the estimated skin of the temporal region, the incision is continued in a caudad direction following the contour marking of the rim of the helix. At the cephalad aspect of the tragus, the incision follows the rim, or edge of the tragus. At the caudad border of the tragus, the incision comes through the deepest portion of the tragus-antitragus notch between the caudad border of the tragus and the cephalad border of the antitragus and continues in a semilunar line following the contour of the junction of the lobule of the ear with the cheek (Fig. 4–6). The incision of the rim of the tragus is carried down to the tragus cartilage. The skin and subcutaneous fat are removed from the external (anterior) surface of the tragal cartilage (see Fig. 4–6), proceeding to a depth that is level with the subcutaneous elevation of the skin of the cheek.

Excision of Pretragal Subcutaneous Fat

After the external (anterior) surface of the tragus is skeletonized, the subdermal dissection of the skin of the cheek is commenced. Elevating the skin at this level leaves a wedge of subcutaneous fat in the pretragal region (Fig. 4–7). To accentuate a sculptured tragus at closure, this is excised (Fig. 4–8).

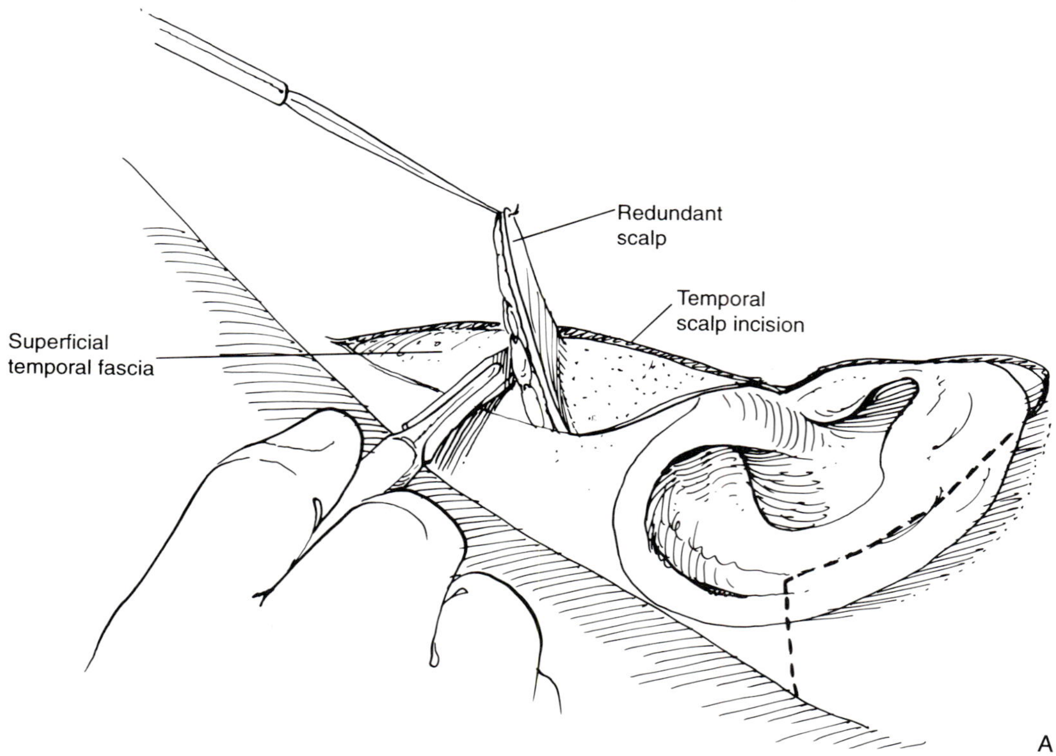

A

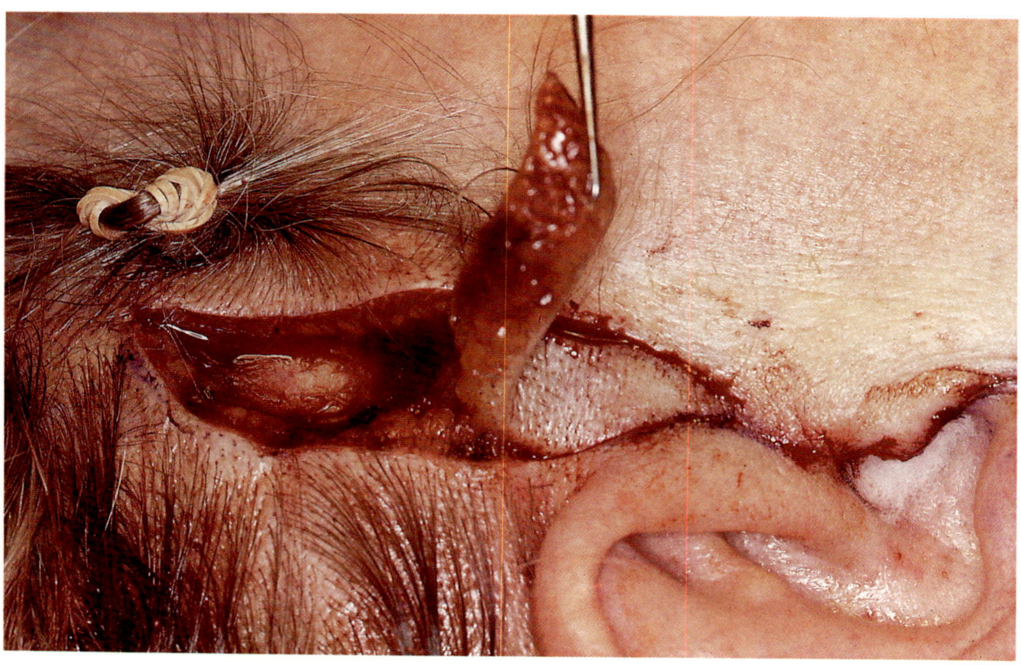

B

Figure 4–2. Excision of the redundant scalp of the temporal region. **A.** Illustration of photograph (B). **B.** Intraoperative.

Figure 4–3. Penetration and opening of the superficial temporal fascia. **A.** Penetration. **B.** Opening, intraoperative.

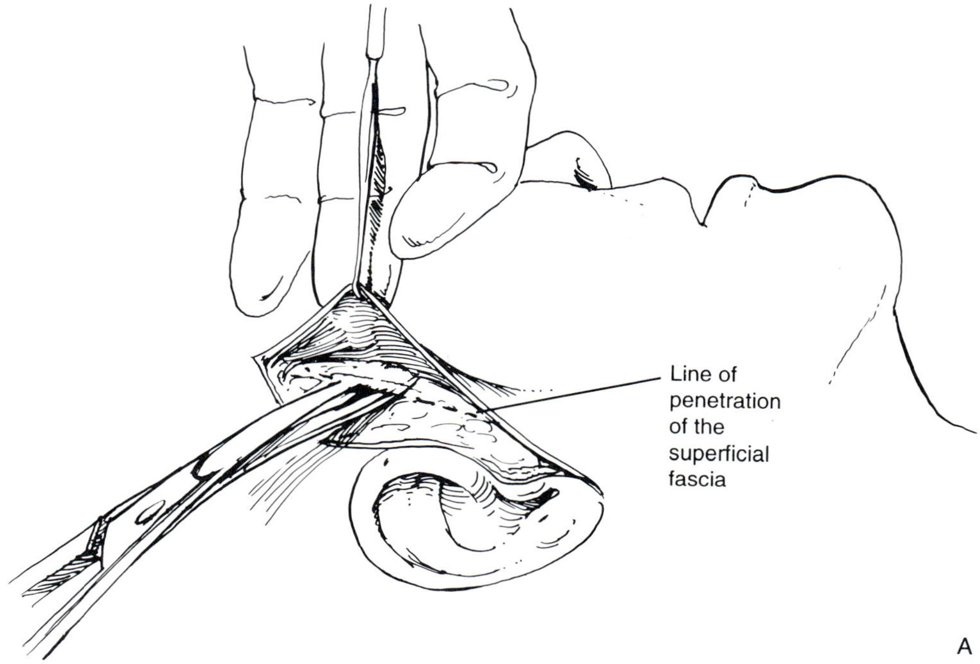

A

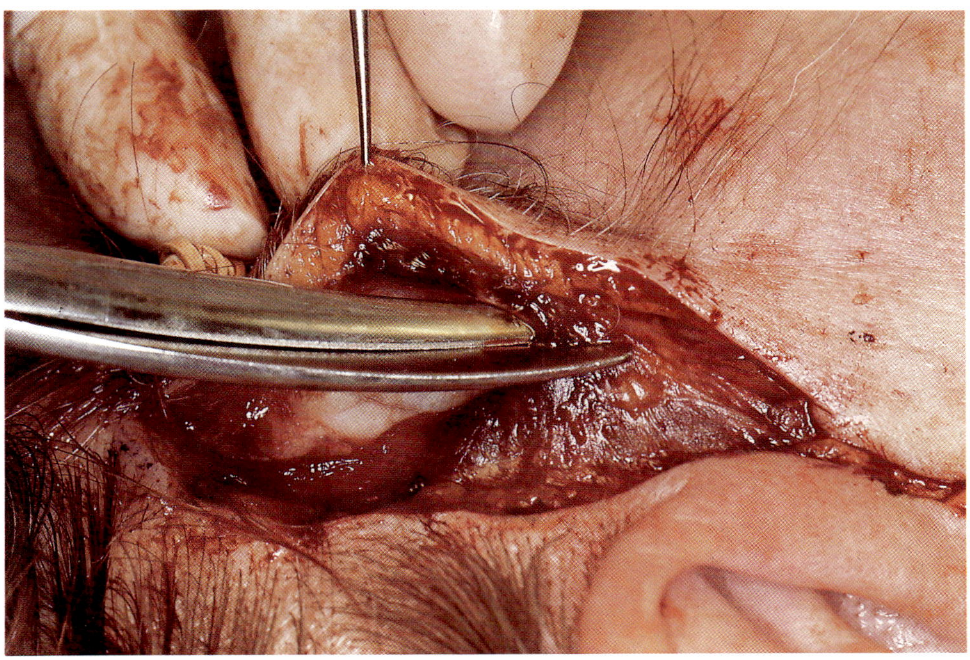

B

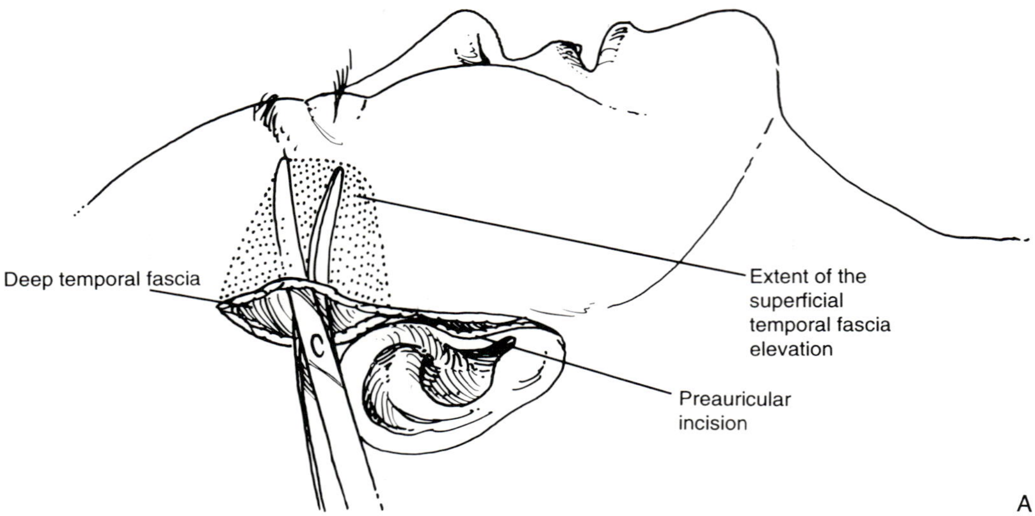

A

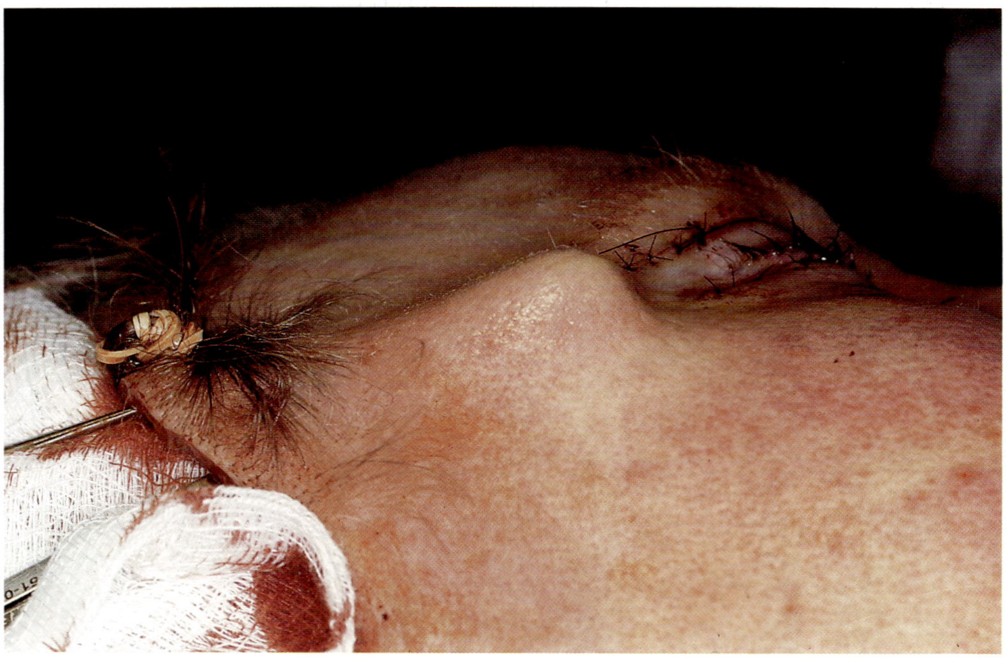

B

Figure 4–4. The extent of the elevation of the superficial temporal fascia. **A.** Illustration of photograph (B). **B.** Intraoperative.

Figure 4–5. Blunt elevation of the superficial temporal fascia.

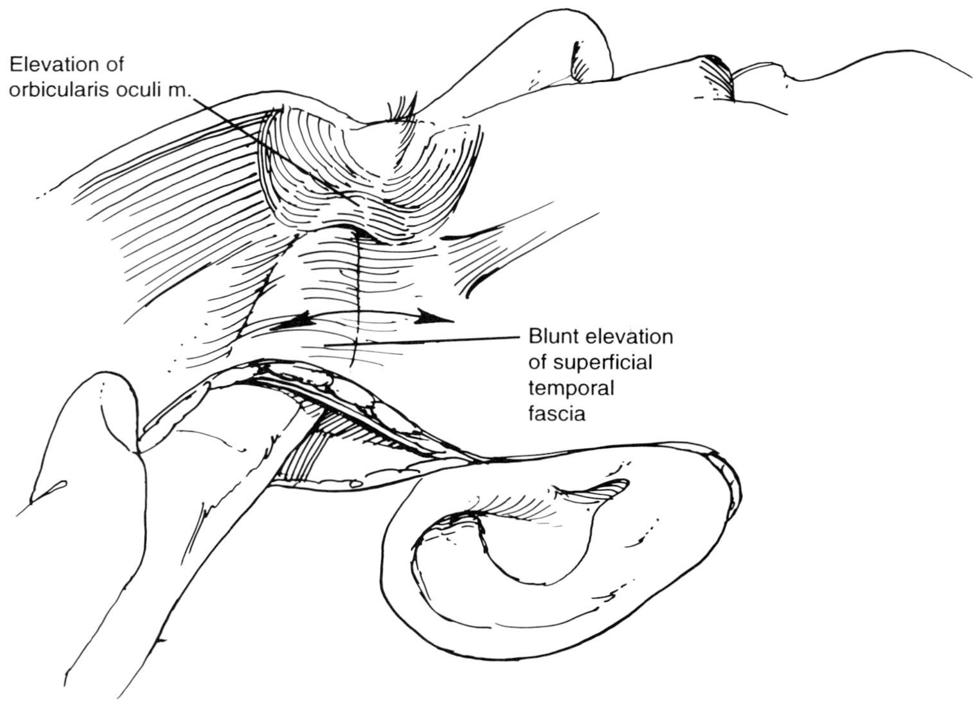

Figure 4–6. The preauricular/tragus incision. **A.** Illustration of photograph (B).

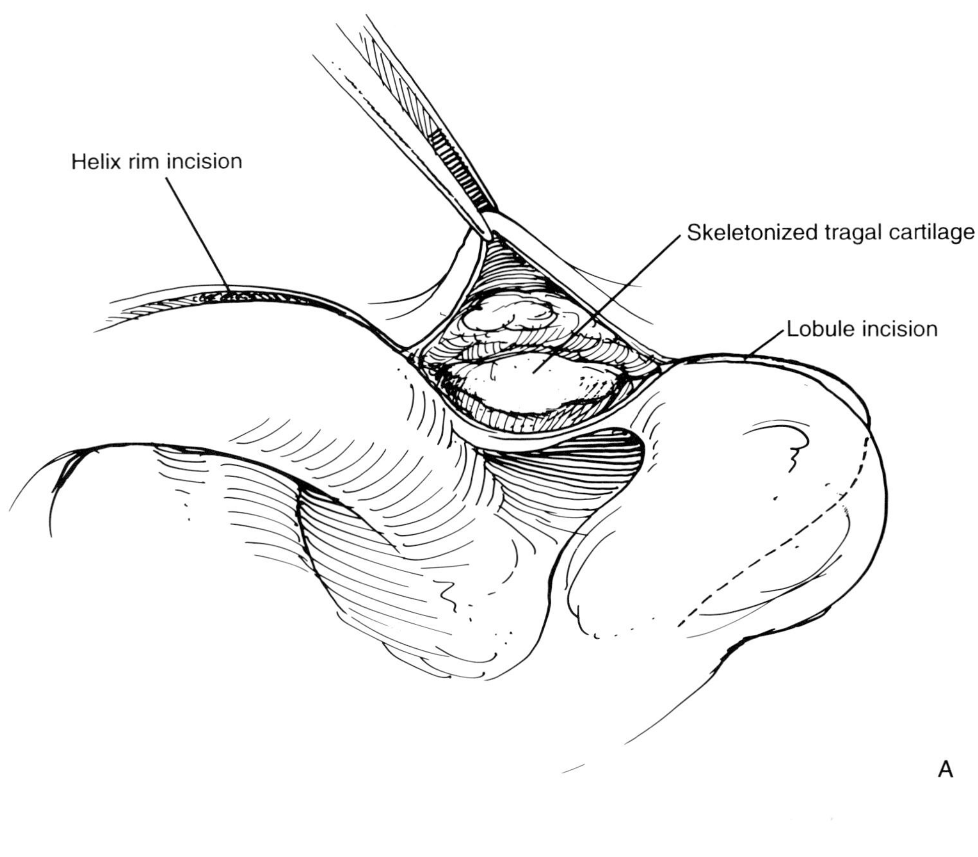

Figure 4–6 (continued) **B.** Intraoperative.

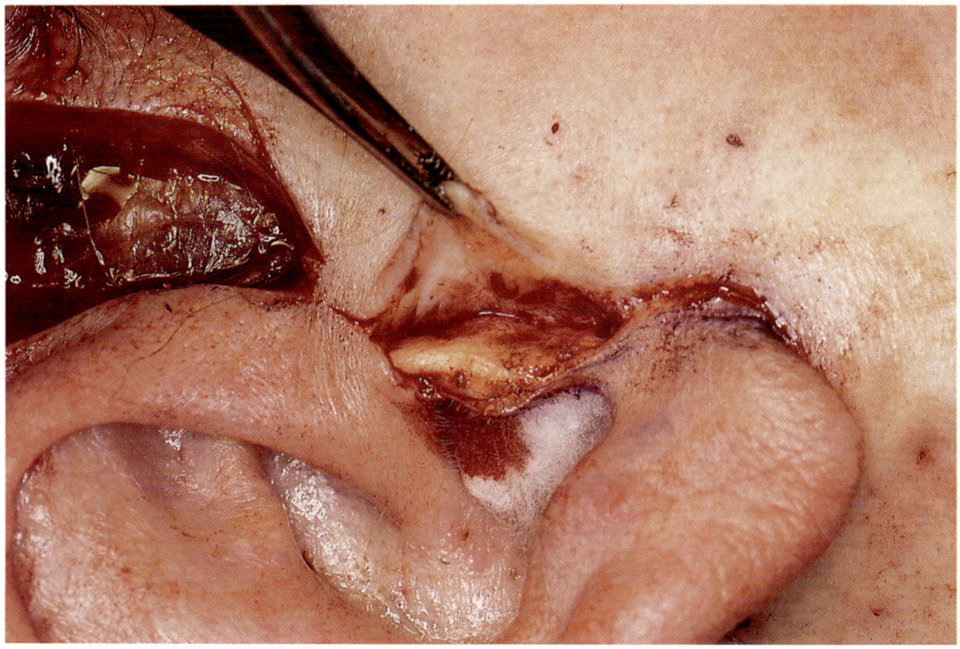

B

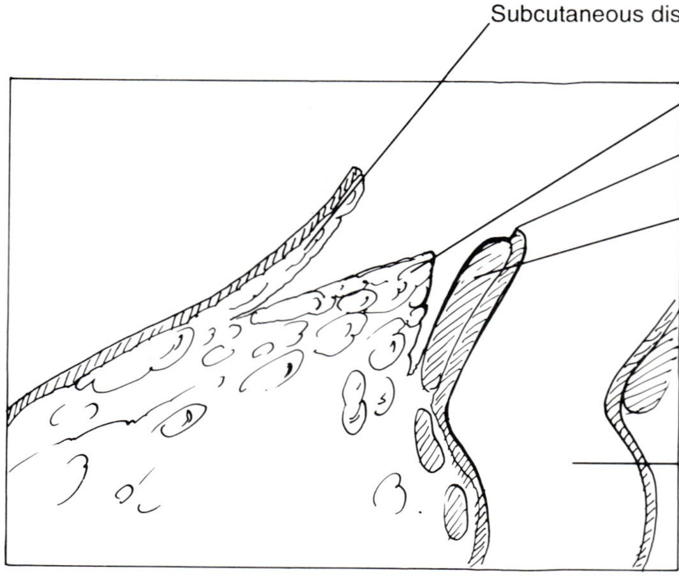

Figure 4–7. Cross section of excess pretragal subcutaneous fat.

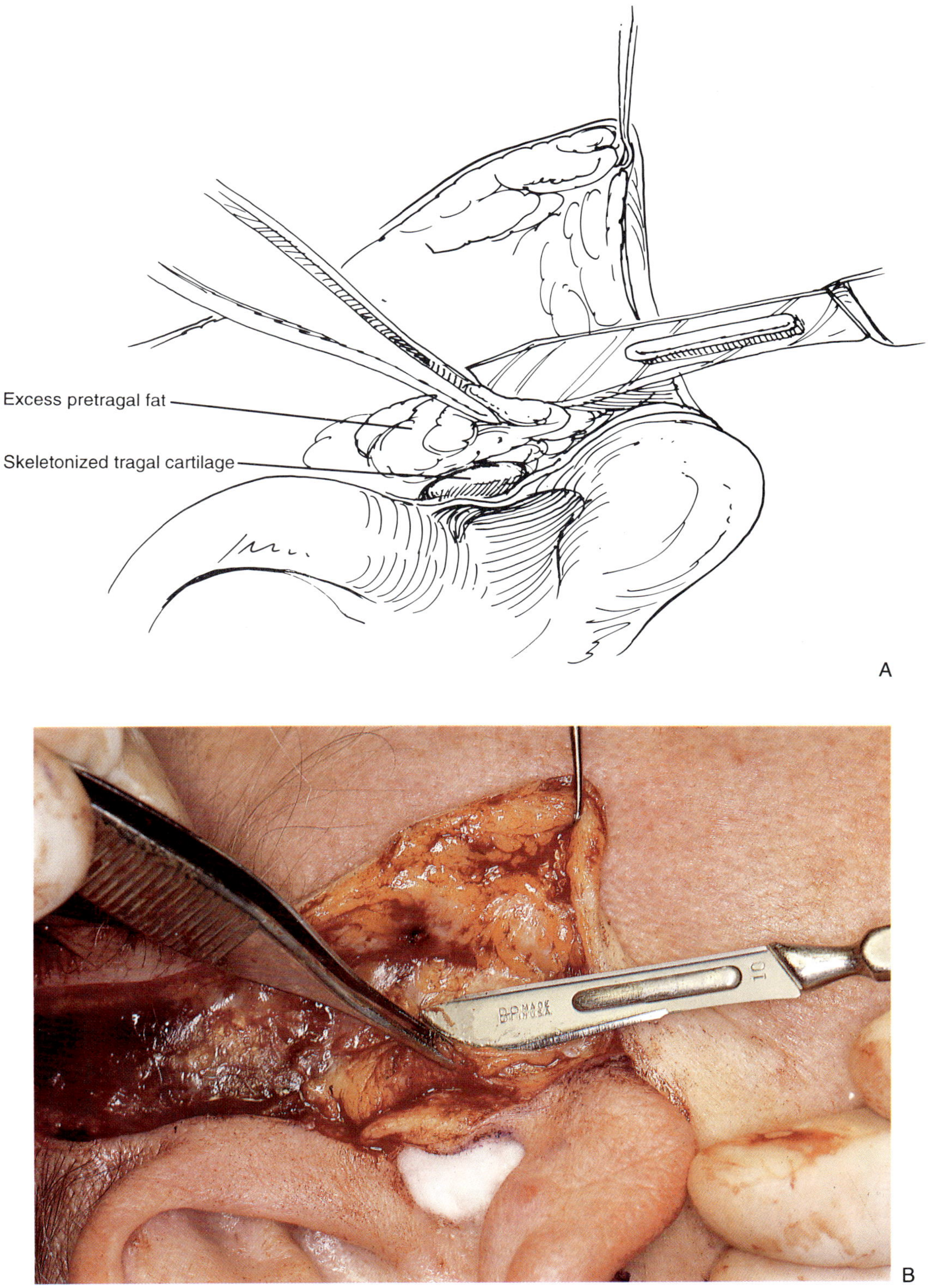

Figure 4–8. Excision of excess pretragal subcutaneous fat. **A.** Illustration of photograph (B). **B.** Intraoperative.

The tragus (anterior surface) and the pretragus region are now prepared to accept the thicker skin of the cheek at wound closure. Subsequently, after the redundant skin of the cheek has been trimmed in preparation for closure of the wound, the skin to be inserted over the skeletonized tragus is defatted and fitted to the tragus rim incision to reproduce a satisfactory sculptured contouring of the tragus (see Chapter 6, Fig. 6–12).

Preliminary Subcutaneous Dissection of the Cheek

After the tragal and pretragal dissection is complete and prior to establishment of the postauricular and occipital incisions, a partial subdermal dissection is commenced in the cheek. This begins below the temporal skin excision and proceeds inferiorly (caudad) to the level of the earlobe junction with the cheek. This phase of the subcutaneous dissection of the cheek is done to partially free the skin, and is accomplished more or less blindly, with the dissection extending medially for a distance of 2.0 to 3.0 cm. No attempt is made at this time to establish the anterior limit of the dissection until the postauricular and posterior cervical flap has been elevated from the underlying tissue. A gauze square* is placed in the wound and the remaining incisions are made.

The Postauricular Incision

The preauricular incision is extended around the attachment of the earlobe to the face, maintaining the incision 1.0 to 1.5 mm peripheral to the crease created by the attachment of the earlobe. The postauricular incision is made as a straight line (Fig. 4–9). The concavity created by the attachment of the earlobe and its skin on the posterior surface of the lobe are preserved as the incision progresses virtually in a straight line beginning at the earlobe's most inferior (caudad) attachment. After passing cephalad to the concavity on the posterior surface of the earlobe, the incision gradually slants anteriorly on the posterior (medial) surface of the concha until at the level of anterior crus of the ear, it is approximately 4 to 5 mm above the postauricular crease (see Chapter 2, Fig. 2–4).

The Occipital Incision

At the level of the anterior (inferior) crus junction with the helix of the ear, the incision proceeds across the narrowest non–hair-bearing area and the area covered by the widest portion of the ear (see Fig. 4–9). Upon passing into the hair-bearing area, the scalpel is moved to a slant, or angled position,

---

*Kendall Vistec, The Kendall Company, Kendall Health Care Products Company, Mansfield, MA 02048.

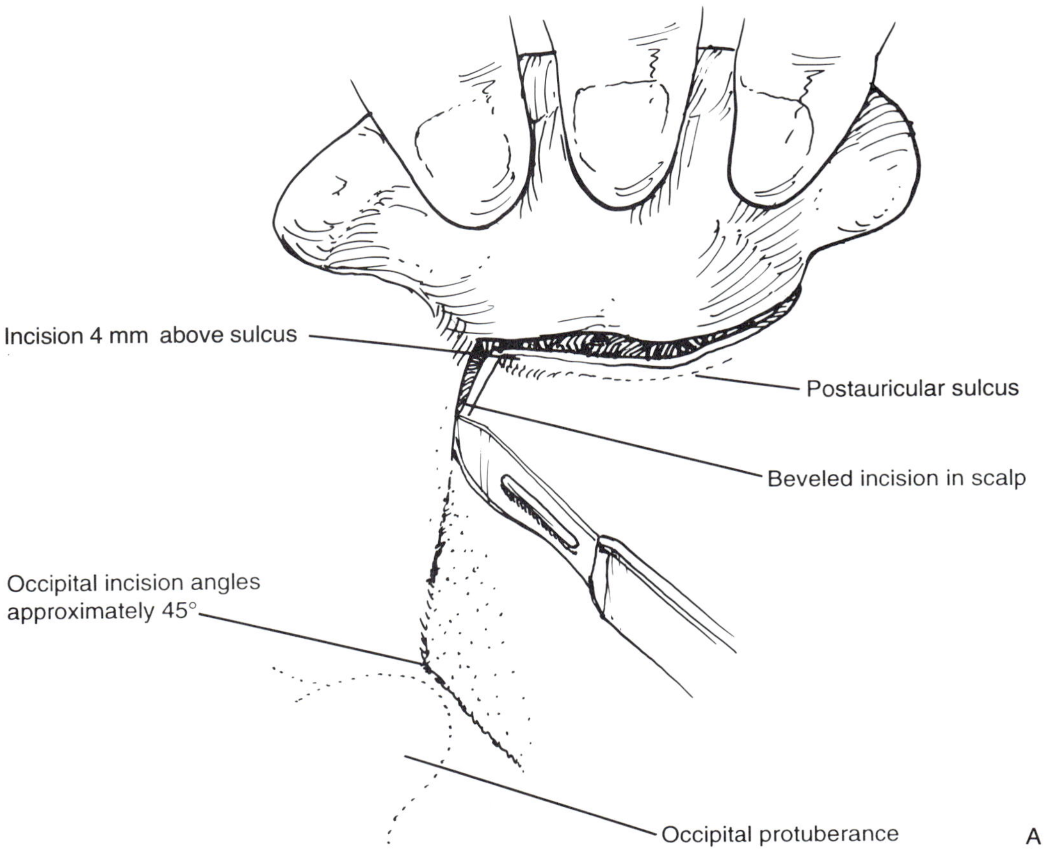

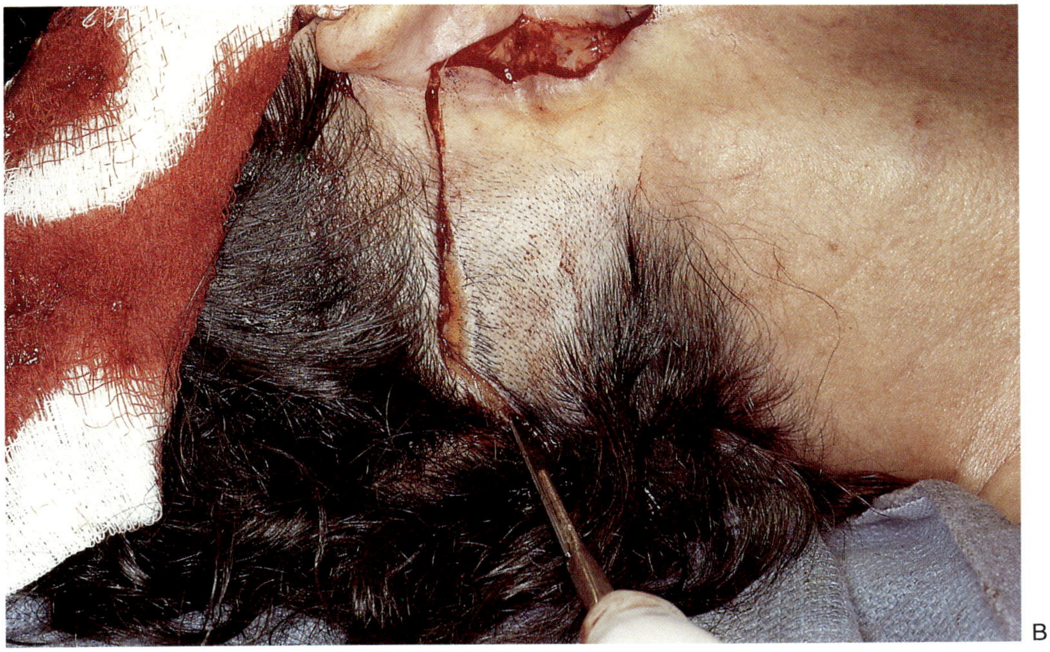

Figure 4–9. Postauricular and occipital incisions. **A.** Illustration of photograph (B). **B.** Intraoperative.

in line with the direction of hair growth to preserve hair follicles. The incision extends posteriorly in a line at right angles to the vertical line of the temporal/ preauricular incision. Just anterior to the occipital protuberance, the incision angles inferiorly (caudad) at approximately a 45-degree angle, extending approximately another 2.0 to 2.5 cm (see Fig. 4–9).

Subcutaneous Dissection of the Postauricular–Posterior Cervical Flap

A sharp skin hook is placed in the postauricular flap in the region of the angle of the incision at the occipital protuberance, and blunt Mayo-type scissors are introduced. The scissors with blunt and sharp dissection easily elevate the hair-bearing tissues. In the region just below the mastoid bone (2.5–3.5 cm caudad of the occipital incision), the superficial and deep fasciae are tightly adherent with no intervening loose areolar tissue. In this area, the skin is thin and very adherent to the underlying fascia. Careful sharp dissection of the adherent area prevents "button-holing"; however, should this occur, the skin flap advancement at closure is usually sufficiently cephalad that it does not interfere with a satisfactory closure.

Beyond the adherent area, the dissection proceeds easily by blunt tip curved Mayo scissor advancement and blade spreading, or advancement with blades of the scissors slightly open. Below the adherent area, approximately 4.0 to 5.0 cm below the earlobe, the great auricular nerve emerges at the posterior border of the sternomastoid muscle (see Chapter 1, Fig. 1–5). With cephalad instrument (single skin hook) traction on the skin and caudad countertraction of the skin by an assistant, the nerve may be elevated and can be transected. Because of this risk, a fiberoptic lighted retractor is introduced after the release of the adherent skin over the mastoid region and the dissection can proceed safely by direct vision. Upon identification of the nerve, or certainty that the dissection is caudad to the emerging nerve, blind dissection can be continued. The caudad limit of the dissection in the posterior cervical region is approximately the level of the cricoid cartilage, but when indicated more caudad. The posterior extent of the dissection is usually along a vertical line dropped from the posterior extent of the occipital incision and at right angles to the occipital incision (Fig. 4–10A, B). Care and caution are necessary to preserve the spinal accessory nerve in this dissection. Fig. 4–10C demonstrates the anterior extent (sternomastoid muscle) of the posterior cervical dissection. This extensive skin elevation in the posterior cervical region allows a smooth drape of the area and aids in the prevention of vertical skin folds in the patient with extensive cutis laxa. Fig. 4–11 shows the extent of the posterior cervical flap dissection. The posterior border of the platysma muscle crossing over the sternomastoid muscle is demonstrated (clamp and scissors).

After the posterior and caudad borders of the posterior cervical skin flap are established, the dissection is directed anteriorly (transversely) across the sternomastoid muscle to join the submental–anterior cervical dissection (see Fig. 4–10C). If the depth of the dissection of the anterior cervical–submental area is subdermal (and the neck has a thin subcutaneous fat layer), the

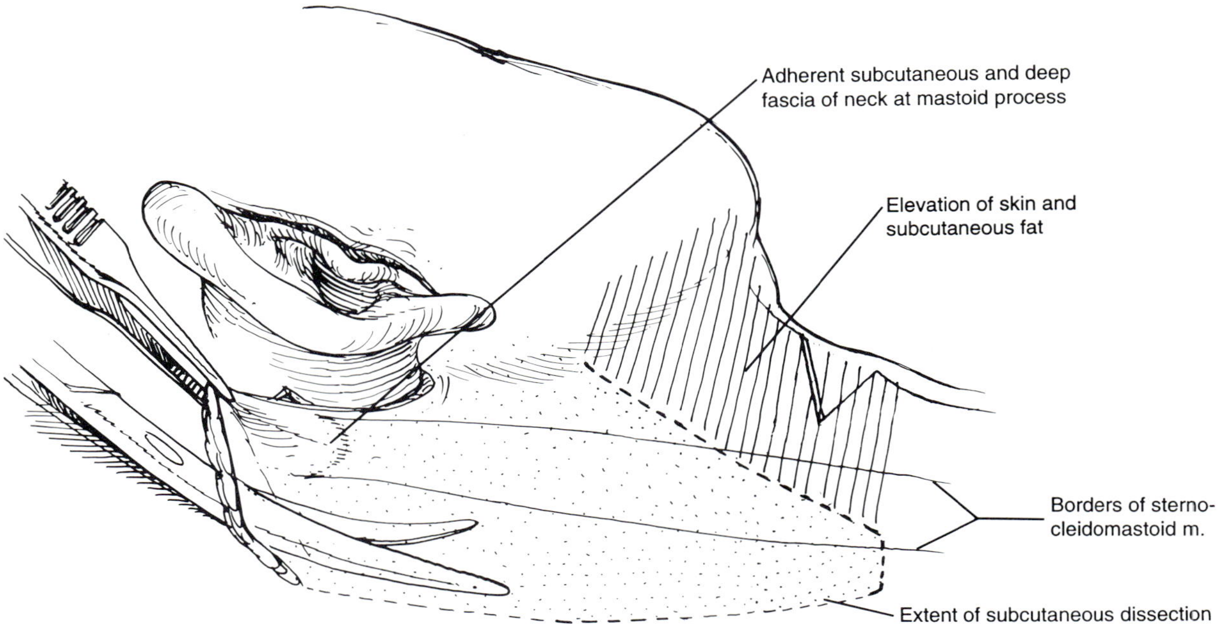

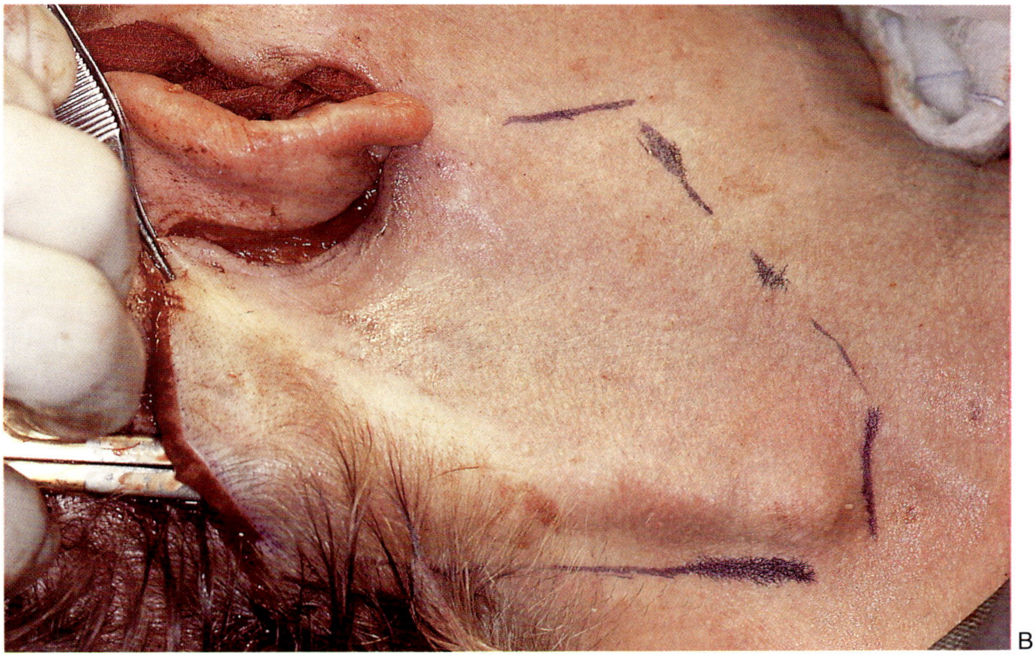

Figure 4–10. Subcutaneous dissection of the postauricular and posterior cervical skin flap. **A.** Illustration of dissection (B). **B.** Posterior extent, intraoperative.

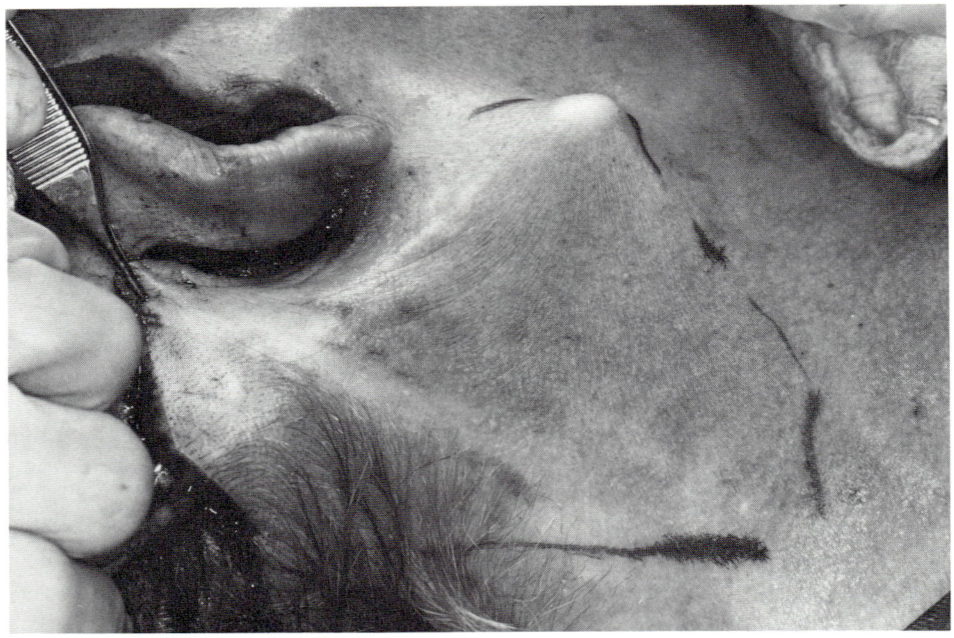

Figure 4–10 (continued) C. Anterior extent, intraoperative.

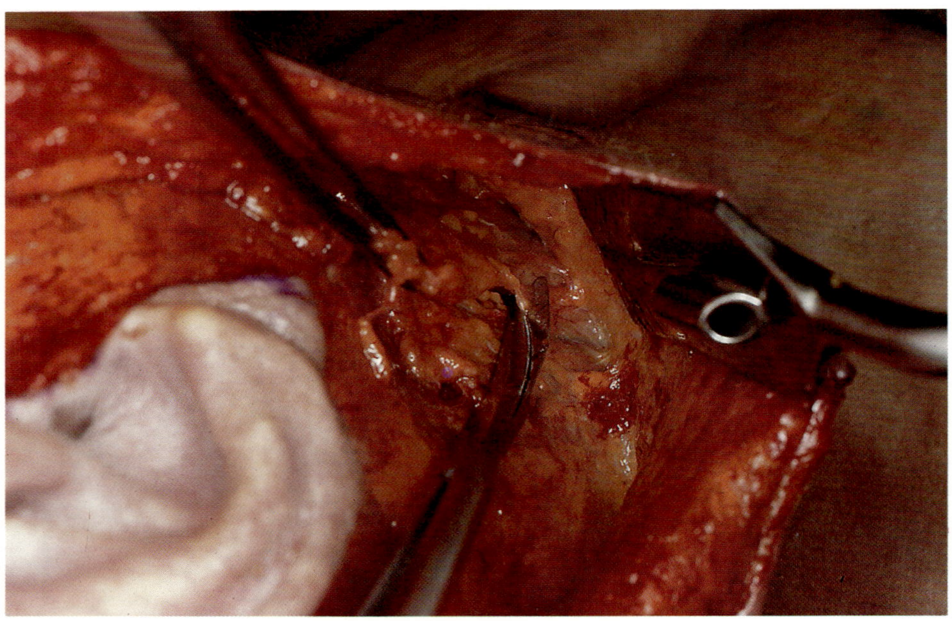

Figure 4–11. The elevated posterior cervical flap. Cephalad to caudad view, intraoperative.

transition at the sternomastoid proceeds at that level. If the anterior cervical/submentum dissection is at the preplatysma muscle level which creates a skin/subcutaneous fat flap, the posterior cervical dissection penetrates from the subdermal skin dissection of the posterior cervical dissection to the preplatysma muscle level of the anterior cervical and submentum region at the posterior border of the sternomastoid muscle. Upon reaching the level of the platysma muscle, the dissection proceeds across the anterior cervical region at the preplatysma level until it joins the preplatysma dissection of the submentum region. That is, the posterior cervical skin flap (subdermal) continues to the midline as a subdermal flap or is converted to a subcutaneous fat–skin flap at the posterior border of the sternomastoid.

With completion of the posterior cervical flap dissection, the area below the ear and over the angle of the mandible is elevated. Single skin hooks are placed in the skin edge about 2.0 cm above the earlobe, anterior and posterior to the earlobe. The posterior cervical subdermal dissection joins the subdermal dissection of the cheek, and the cheek dissection is carried down across the mandible as a subdermal dissection, or at the lower border of the mandible penetrates the subcutaneous fat and joins the subcutaneous fat–skin flap of the neck. The subdermal dissection of the cheek can proceed now to the desired limits.

Subcutaneous Dissection of the Cheek

The borders of the subcutaneous dissection of the periorbital and cheek areas (see Fig. 4–1) extend from the preauricular incision superiorly to a horizontal line at a level approximately 1.0 to 2.0 cm above the zygoma. The subcutaneous dissection overlaps the caudad dissection elevating the superficial temporal fascia. This creates the mesenteric attachment of the skin to the zygomatic arch attachments of the superficial temporal fascia (SMAS) in this region. The orbicularis oculi is partially elevated along its inferiolateral and inferior border. At the posterior border of the malar eminence (see Fig. 4–1), the anterior border of the subcutaneous dissection drops inferiorly (caudad) along a line that will meet the posterior border of the platysma muscle at the inferior border of the mandible (see Fig. 4–1).

The release of the postauricular–posterior cervical skin flap, which has joined the anterior cervical–submental flap, provides the relaxation to extend the moderate subcutaneous dissection made at the time of the skin incision to the stated borders.

Approximately 1.5 to 2.0 cm above the lower border of the mandible posteriorly (see Fig. 4–1), the subdermal dissection of the cheek is angled toward the jowl area. This joins the submental and anterior cervical dissection at the inferior border of the mandible at the subdermal level or the subcutaneous fat–skin flap level. If indicated, the mandibular ligament attachments are released. The subdermal release of the skin in this manner will permit satisfactory advancement of the skin flap and will provide a smooth drape of the skin over the mandible line.

The decision of whether to create a more extensive release of the skin over the mandible or to keep the SMAS–subcutaneous fat–skin complex intact is made in general on evaluation of the changes presented by the patient. If the aging changes are minimal in the face and neck and the patient is young, a SMAS advancement of the cheeks without release of the skin over the border of the mandible is sufficient. With increased age and more extensive skin relaxation of the jowl area and neck, and in the thinner individual, the release of the mandibular ligaments and the skin from the SMAS over the mandible permits a better bidirectional drape of the skin. The skin overlying the mandible and the neck (anterior and posterior cervical flaps) can be pulled in a more posterior cephalad direction while the SMAS is pulled in a more cephalad posterior direction (see Chapter 6, Fig. 6–1).

At this juncture, the "mesentery" of the superficial temporal fascia is left intact, and will be released "as necessary" at the time of the wound closure. Fig. 4–12 demonstrates the extent of the subdermal dissection of the cheek and the elevated superficial temporal fascia with the intervening mesentery intact.

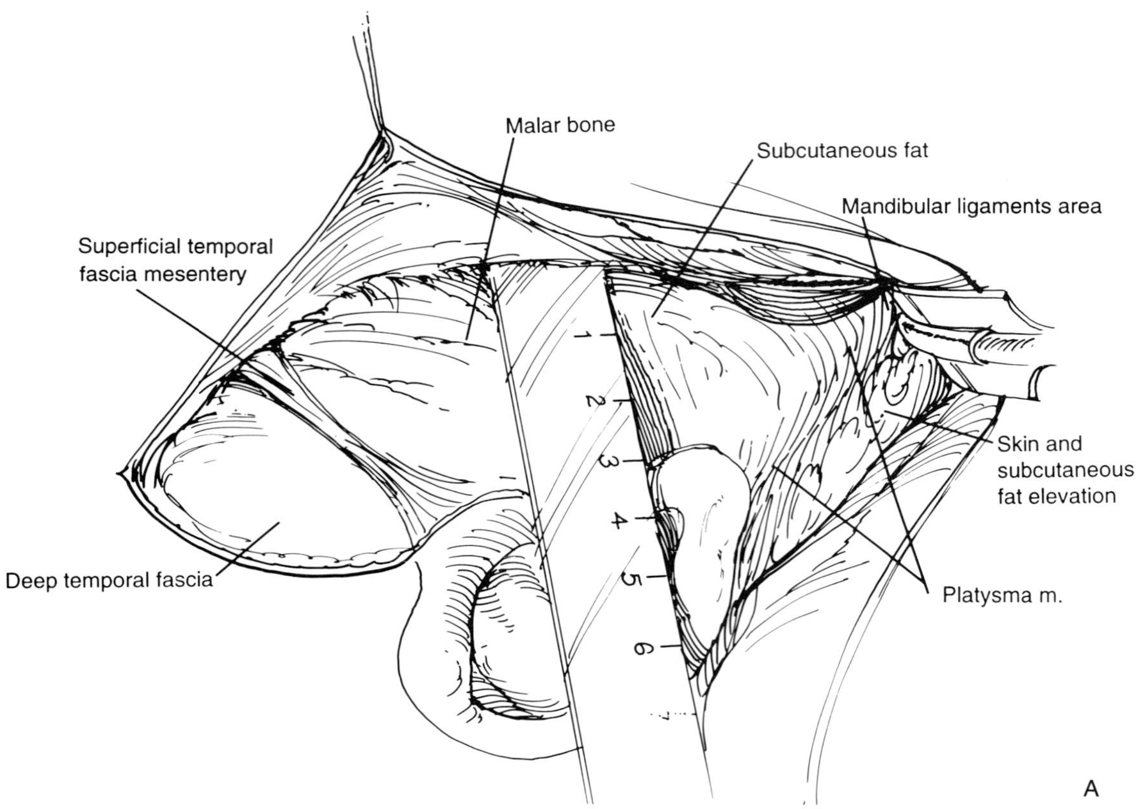

Figure 4–12. Subdermal dissection of the cheek and elevated superficial temporal fascia. **A.** Illustrations of photograph (B) and (C).

Figure 4–12 (continued) **B.** Cadaver. **C.** Intraoperative.

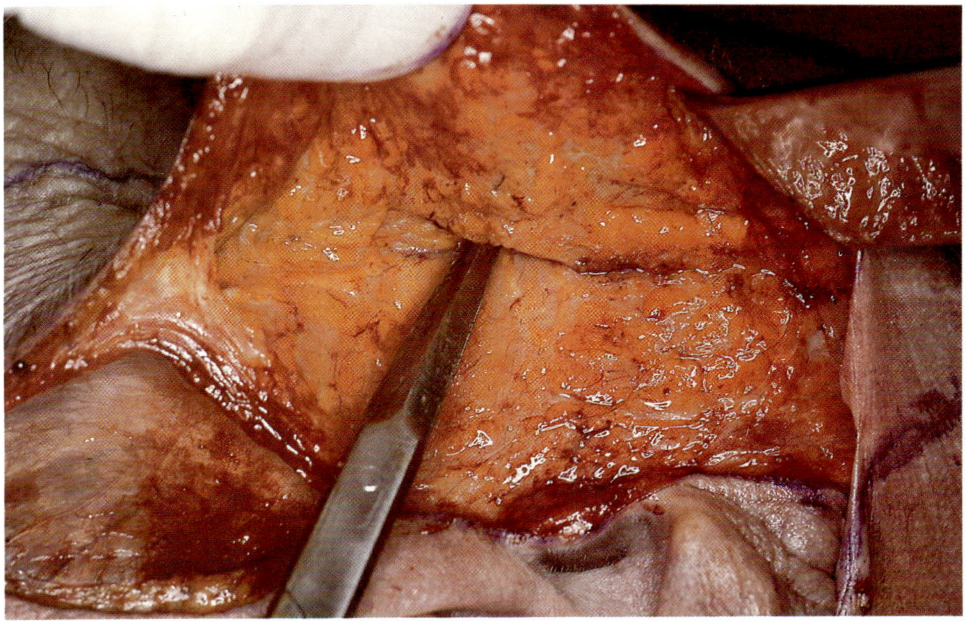

B

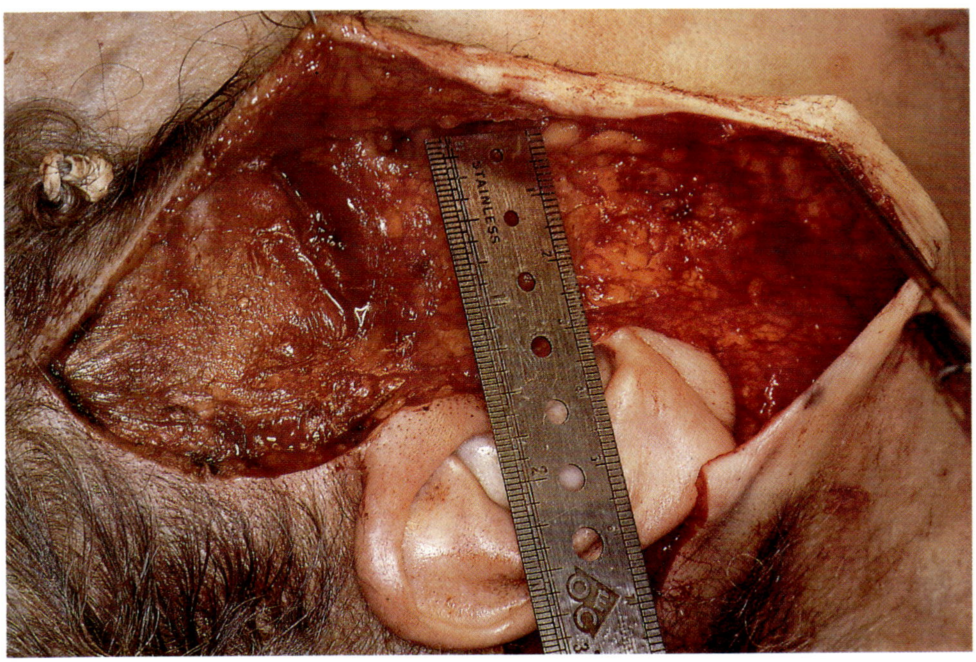

C

FIVE

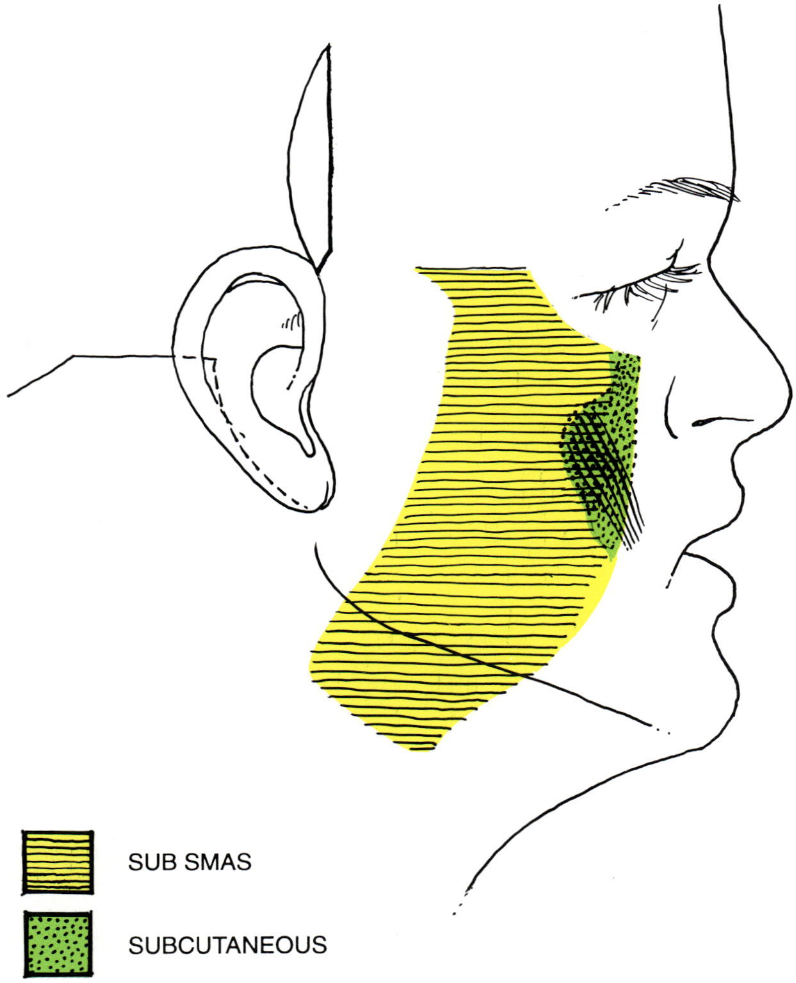

The Mobilization and Advancement of the Cheek SMAS

The objective of the SMAS elevation and advancement, or reconstruction of the attenuated SMAS, is to provide a significant reduction of the nasolabial fold crease and to reestablish a smooth jawline. If this is not achieved to a sufficient degree in the upper part of the face to equal the results achievable in the neck, the cheeks (face) may appear to "overhang" the jawline and neck.

To accomplish the desired results, SMAS elevation anteriorly should extend to the nasolabial fold. Skoog[1] stated this in his original publication. He recognized the necessity of reaching the nasolabial fold, but seemed to believe that the penetration and partial release, rather than a complete release of the tissues, were sufficient to achieve a satisfactory (and lasting) improvement of the nasolabial fold crease. Subsequent evolution of the Skoog procedure has been more a matter of extensive release of the tissues in reaching the nasolabial fold than, in Skoog's description, a penetration to the nasolabial fold and spreading of the scissors beyond the anterior border of masseter muscle with some of the intervening tissue remaining intact. The intervening tissue connections to the dermis have been described as ligaments originating either from the platysma muscle (anterior platysma–cutaneous) or from the masseter muscle (masseter-cutaneous) (see Chapter 1). The release of this adherent region does produce a more mobile flap, which permits its complete advancement to a new site without any tethering. Experience with extensive mobilization of the SMAS to the nasolabial fold does seem to produce a superior result compared to a partial release.

Improvement of the nasolabial fold and its inferior extension to the mandible is the objective of the SMAS dissection. This is accomplished best by releasing all tissues to the nasolabial fold that may restrain a satisfactory advancement necessary to reduce the fold. The SMAS elevation is commenced anterior to the thicker, and more strongly adherent parotid-masseteric fascia. This brings the line of support for the nasolabial fold closer to the defect (a deep nasolabial fold), and it provides a strong purchase for the advanced SMAS. Also, if the dissection extends to the nasolabial fold, the dissection time is reduced when compared with the time needed for SMAS elevation, which begins more posterior in the preauricular area of the parotid-masseteric fascia.

Table 5–1 outlines the intraoperative sequence of the SMAS and cheek dissection.

Fig. 5–1 illustrates the sub-SMAS and infraorbital subcutaneous areas of the dissection.

The course of the dissection of the SMAS in the cheek is divided into the zygomatic, buccal, and mandibular zones. Each zone represents a quadrilat-

Table 5–1. The Intraoperative Sequence of the Mobilization and Advancement of the SMAS and Cheek

1. Penetration of the SMAS
2. Mobilization of the zygomatic (nasolabial fold) zone
3. Mobilization of the buccal zone
4. Mobilization of the mandibular zone
5. Posterior-cephalad advancement of the SMAS
6. Closure of the advanced SMAS
7. Trimming of the redundant SMAS

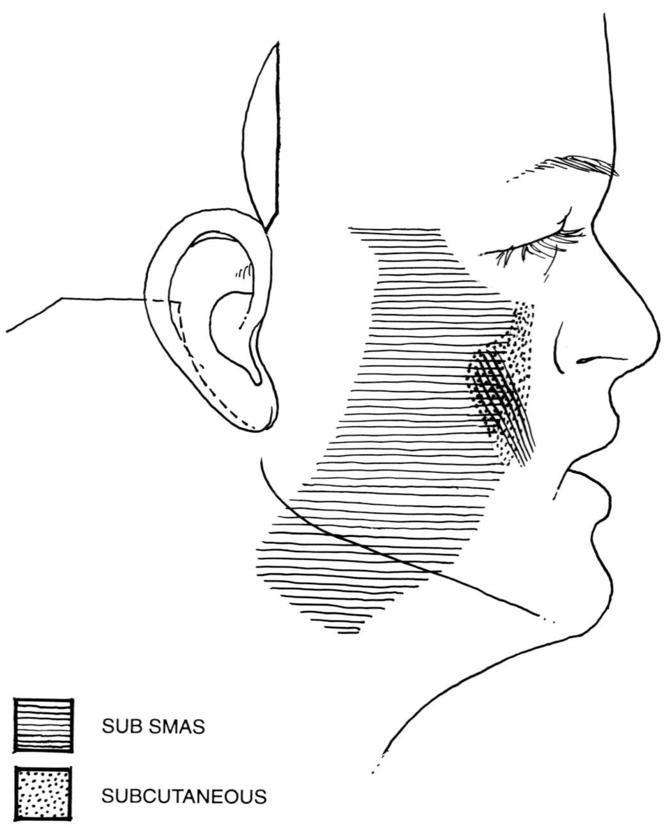

Figure 5–1. The sub-SMAS and the subcutaneous dissection of the cheek.

eral area which presents different features that require recognition and special handling (Fig. 5–2).

The significant anatomical structures of the zygomatic segment of the sub-SMAS dissection include the orbicularis oculi muscle, the malar prominence and the zygomaticus major and minor muscles, and a branch of the zygomatic nerve (see Chapter 1, Fig. 1–2). The buccal branch of the facial nerve and the nerve supply to the zygomaticus major muscle lie deep to the zygomaticus major muscle and under the deep fascia of the head. If the dissection of this area approaches from the malar prominence at an angle that is more or less perpendicular to the nasolabial fold, the plane of dissection will be superficial to the zygomatic major muscle and the facial nerve branches protected. Stating this another way, if the dense tissues in the malar region are freed in the dome [under surface (deep) of the superficial fascia] of the

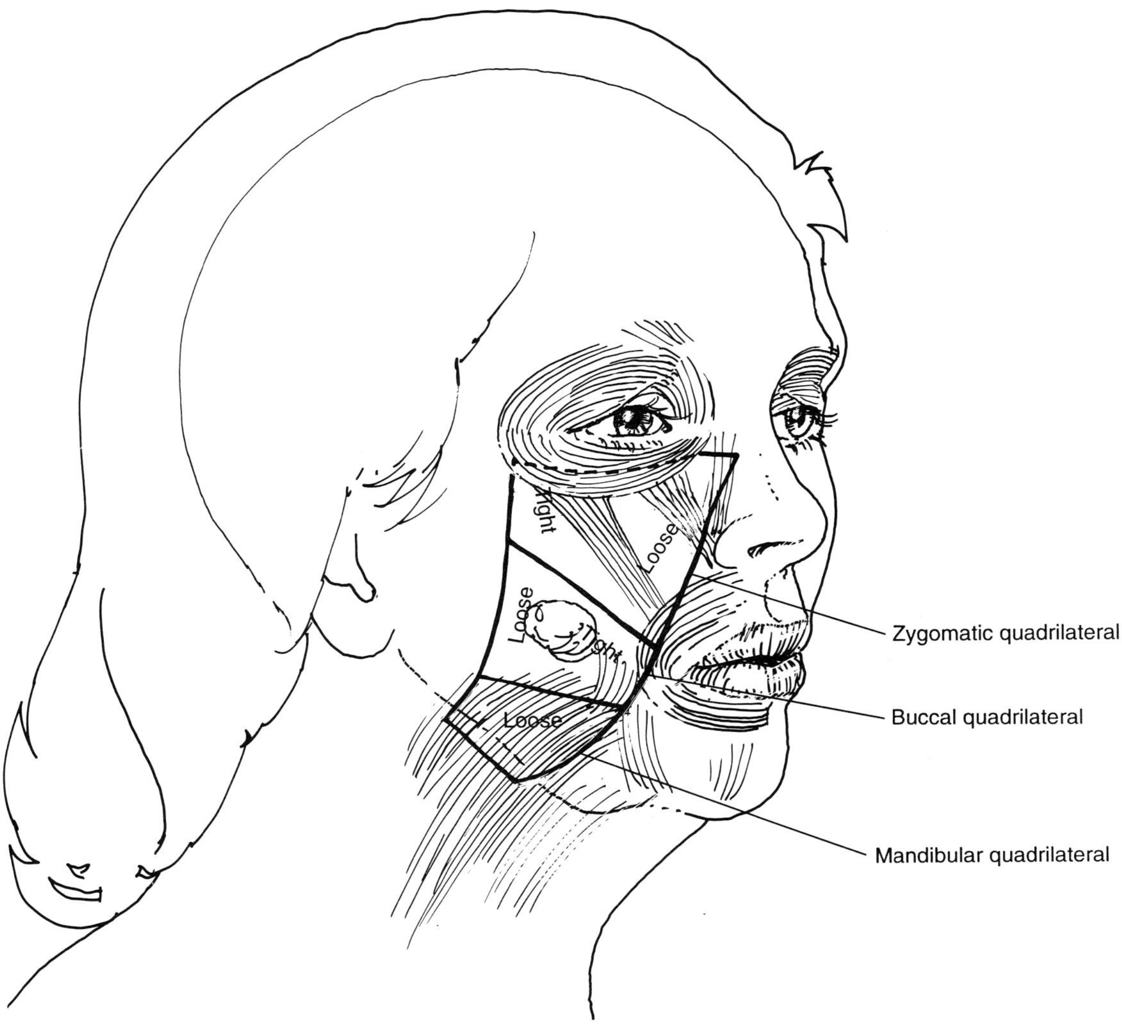

Figure 5–2. The sub-SMAS and infraorbital dissection of the cheek: the zones and the degree of tissue adherence in the zone.

dissection, the plane proceeds into the subcutaneous tissues of the infraorbital area anterior (medial) to the zygomaticus major muscle. If the approach in the zygomatic segment is from a more lateral, or inferior direction, the dissection proceeds at a sub-SMAS level, which (more often than not) advances deep to the zygomaticus major muscle. This can imperil the zygomatic and the buccal branch of the facial nerve. If the dissection does drop deep to the zygomaticus major muscle, this becomes clear almost immediately and a more superficial approach is established. Identifying the origin of the zygomaticus muscle on the malar prominence can be used as the guide to the nasolabial fold. However, as long as the dissection continues in the "dome" of the release over the malar prominence, or more superficial than deep, actual identification of the zygomaticus major muscle is not a requirement.

Anterior (medial) and superficial to the zygomaticus major muscle and extending to and across the inferior orbital rim to the nasal process of the maxillary bone is a "safe" area (see Chapter 1, Fig. 1–2). After crossing the zygomaticus major muscle superficially, the dissection is in the subcutaneous fat of the infraorbital area (see Fig. 5–1).

The important anatomical structures of the buccal sub-SMAS segment (Fig. 5–2) are observed anterior to the parotid gland and include the buccal branch of the facial nerve, the parotid duct deep to the nerve branches, and the buccal fat pad. The transverse facial artery is deep to the "web" of facial nerve branches and rarely visualized.

The lower zone of the SMAS elevation in the cheek (mandibular) (Fig. 5–2) is over the parotid gland and beneath the platysma muscle. The branches of the facial nerve in the area are the marginal mandibular (submandibular branch) and the cervical. The marginal mandibular branch, a single branch, supplies the quadratus labii inferioris muscle and the mentalis muscle of the lower lip. The cervical branch supplies the platysma muscle. Injury to the marginal mandibular branch (submandibular muscle) results in temporary or permanent loss of the lower-lip function.

Penetration of the SMAS

After the subdermal dissection of the cheek has reached anteriorly to the proposed line of penetration to the sub-SMAS plane, the penetration to the deep plane is achieved by placing upward and posterior traction with a single skin hook retractor in the skin edge (Fig. 5–3A, B). With the fingers on the external surface of the skin, the cheek tissues are pulled toward the operator. This presents the proposed line of penetration of the SMAS at the anterior extent of the subdermal dissection. This "tents" the SMAS and rolls it over upon itself. With either a knife blade (number 10) or scissors (blunt tip curved Mayo-type)*, the "tented" area is scored lightly in a direction tangential to the skin until penetration has occurred and the undersurface (deep) of the SMAS appears (Fig. 5–3C, D).

The deep surface of the SMAS is recognizable as a distinct and deeper fascial plane. At this distance anterior to the preauricular incision, the SMAS

*The dissection in Chapter 5 employs the core set of instruments listed in Chapter 3.

Figure 5–3. The penetration of the SMAS of the cheek. **A.** Cross section of the penetration of the SMAS and subcutaneous fat. **B.** Illustration of photographs (C) and (D).

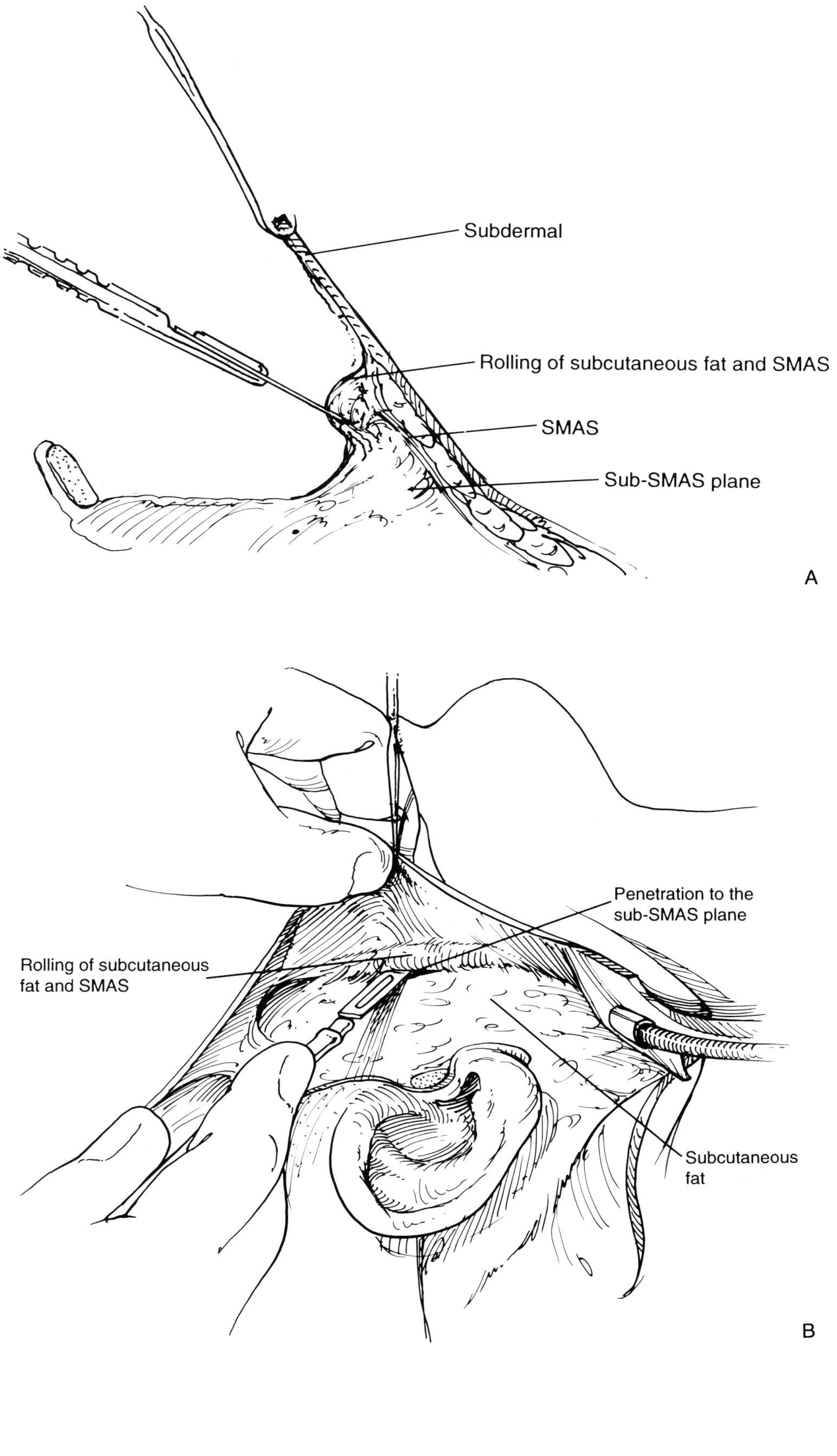

Figure 5–3 (continued) **C.** Cadaver. **D.** Intraoperative.

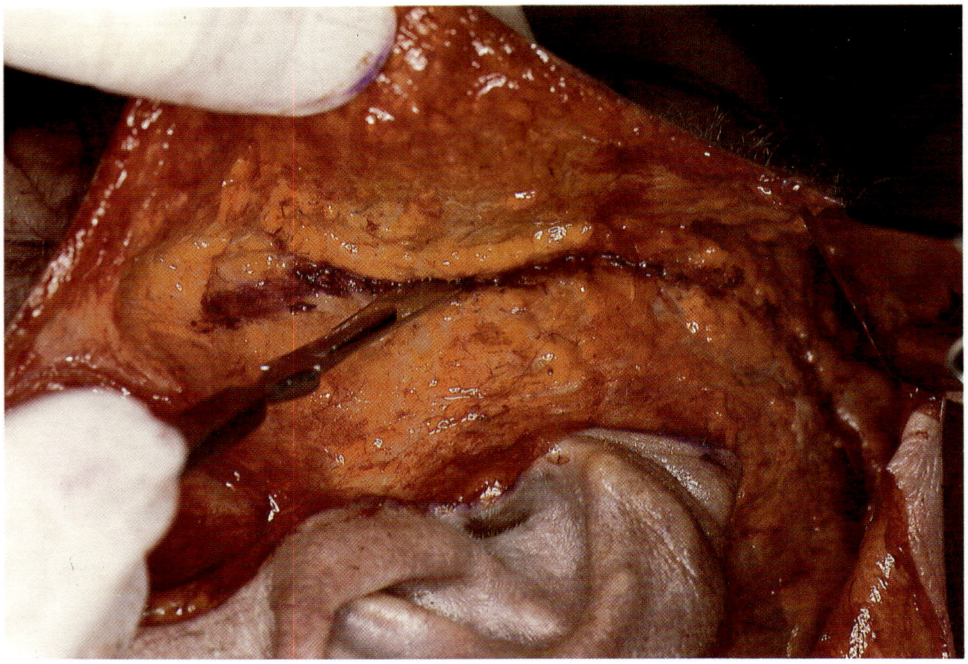

C

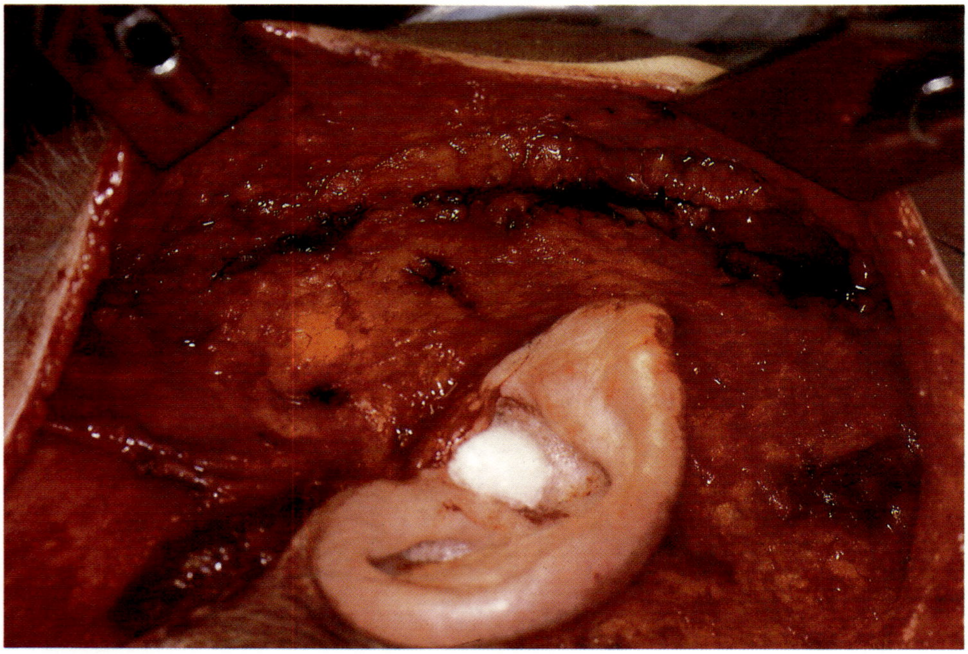

D

and the deep fascia can be easily separated. The deep surface of the SMAS is a denser collagen fiber layer that appears shinier and ranges in color from a suggestive silvery-white characteristic of fascial planes to the yellow(ish) color of fat when the density of the collagen and the fascia plane is not well developed. The posterior border of the SMAS is elevated by extending the point of penetration of the SMAS superiorly and inferiorly to the zygoma and to the submandibular area, respectively.

After the posterior border of the SMAS is elevated from the deep fascia (at the point of penetration or medial edge of the SMAS penetration), the dissection proceeds medially in the direction of or at the level of the malar prominence. Shortly thereafter, just below the malar prominence a single perforating branch of the transverse facial artery is transected. After this vessel is secured, further bleeding in the sub-SMAS plane usually is minimal.

Elevation of the Zygomatic (Nasolabial Fold) Zone

Once the sub-SMAS plane has been identified and its superior and inferior limits established, the dissection proceeds to develop the anterior or medial border of the sub-SMAS dissection. In establishing the superior and inferior limits of the portion of the SMAS to be elevated, 1.0 to 1.5 cm of the SMAS has been elevated in a medial (anterior) direction. The upper zone (zygomatic nasolabial fold quadrilateral) (see Fig. 5–2) at its posterior (malar) aspect is firmly adherent over the malar process. The dense tissue plane, or zygomatic ligament (McGregors's patch), is separated with scissors and strong finger pressure. The sub-SMAS in this area is well defined and as in most all areas of the separation of the SMAS and the deep fascia of the head, the tissue transection is done in the "dome" of the elevated SMAS (deep surface of the SMAS) a few millimeters posterior (lateral) to the adherent superficial and deep fasciae. Approximately 5 to 10 mm of the inferior border of the orbicularis oculi muscle (Fig. 5–4A) is elevated as the dissection proceeds medially to an imaginary vertical line drawn from the junction of the nasolabial fold and the alar base of the nose to the inferior orbital rim (see Fig. 5–1). On the sub-SMAS (deep) surface, the orbicularis oculi fibers are visible.

Over the inferior-anterior portion of the malar prominence, the fibers of the zygomaticus major muscle can be identified (see Fig. 5–4). The zygomaticus major muscle proceeds in an oblique direction to attach just lateral to the corner of the mouth and represents the lower border of the zygomatic quadrilateral. Proceeding from the superior border of the quadrilateral (inferior border of the elevated orbicularis oculi muscle), the SMAS is elevated anteriorly and inferiorly. Anterior to the firm, dense tissues over the malar bone prominence, the dissection becomes easier as it reverts from the sub-SMAS plane back to the subcutaneous plane (see Fig. 5–1). The release of the tissues external (superficial) to the zygomaticus major muscle and cephalad (superior) to the zygomaticus major muscle (the SMAS) from the malar prominence to the nasolabial fold or slightly below it provides a satisfactory release for an optimal advancement.

As stated previously, if the strong, tightly adherent SMAS over the malar prominence is elevated first and the dissection then proceeds from this point

Figure 5–4. The zygomatic zone dissection: the zygomaticus major muscle and the subcutaneous dissection medial to the zygomaticus major muscle. **A.** Illustration of photographs (B) and (C). **B.** Cadaver (zygomaticus major muscle with superficial fascia removed).

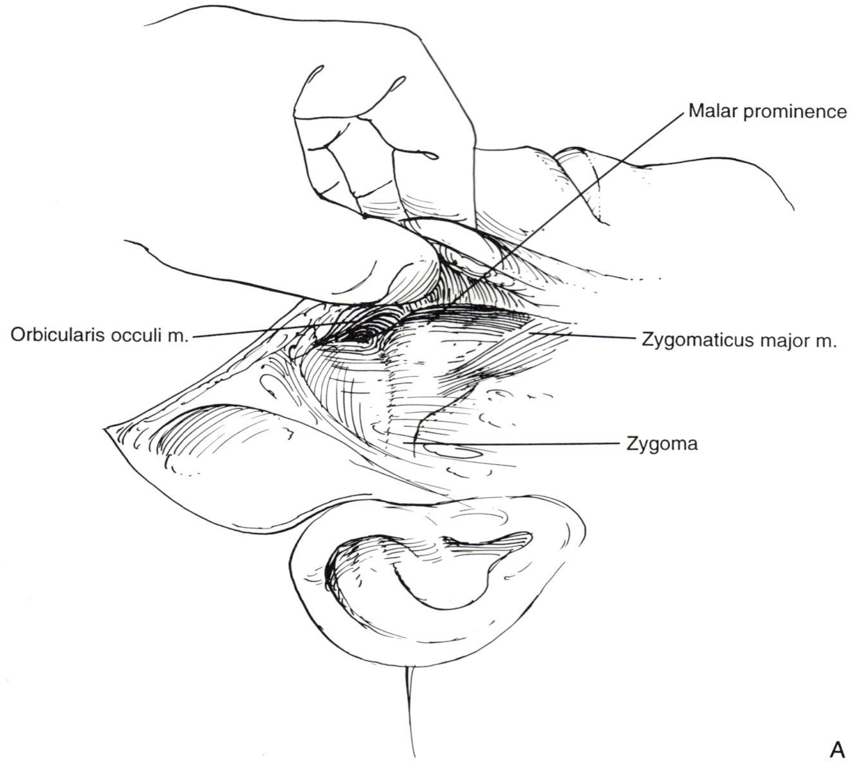

A

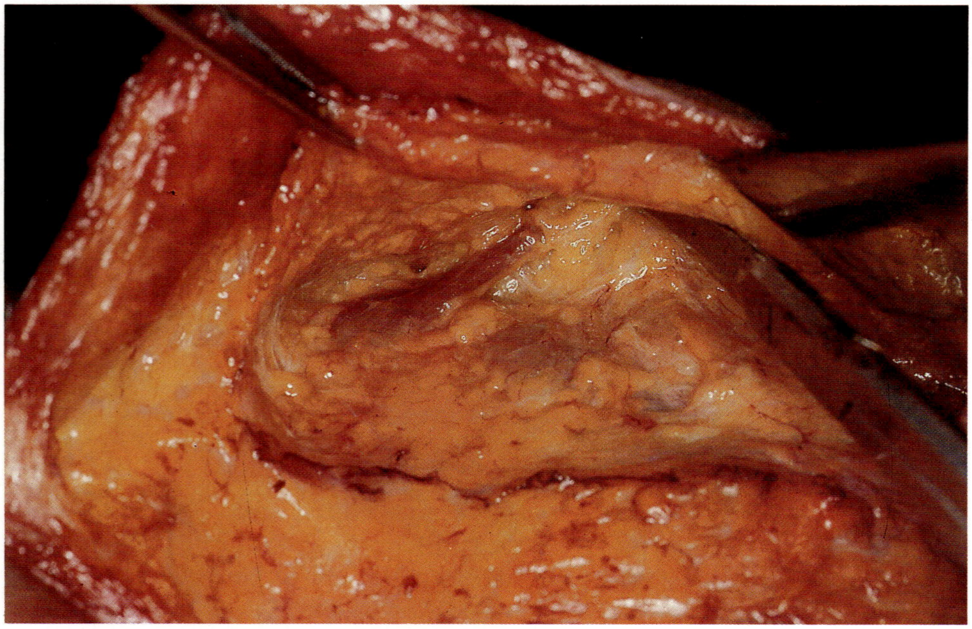

B

Figure 5–4 (continued) **C.** Intraoperative (zygomaticus major muscle outlined in methylene blue; epinephrine dilution 1:400,000). **D.** Intraoperative (scissor tips on the zygomaticus major muscle; epinephrine dilution 1:100,000).*

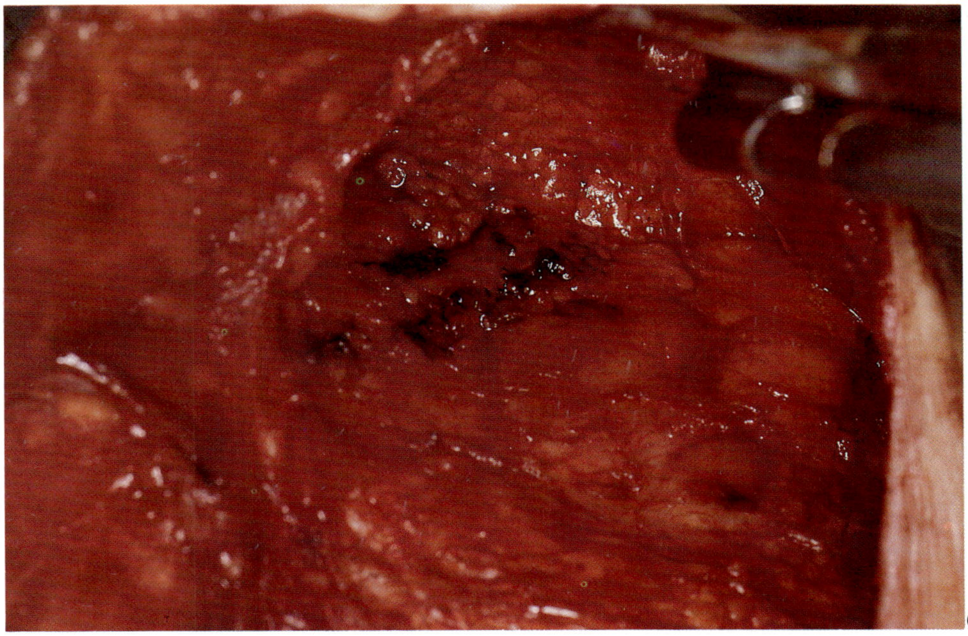

C

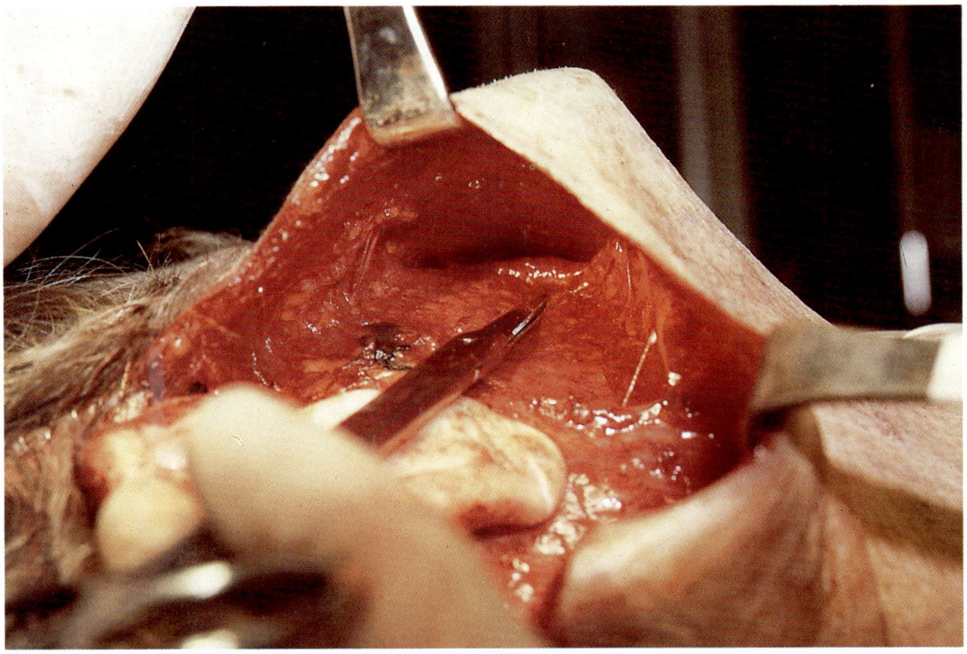

D

*Epinephrine dilution of 1:100,000 for demonstration purposes.

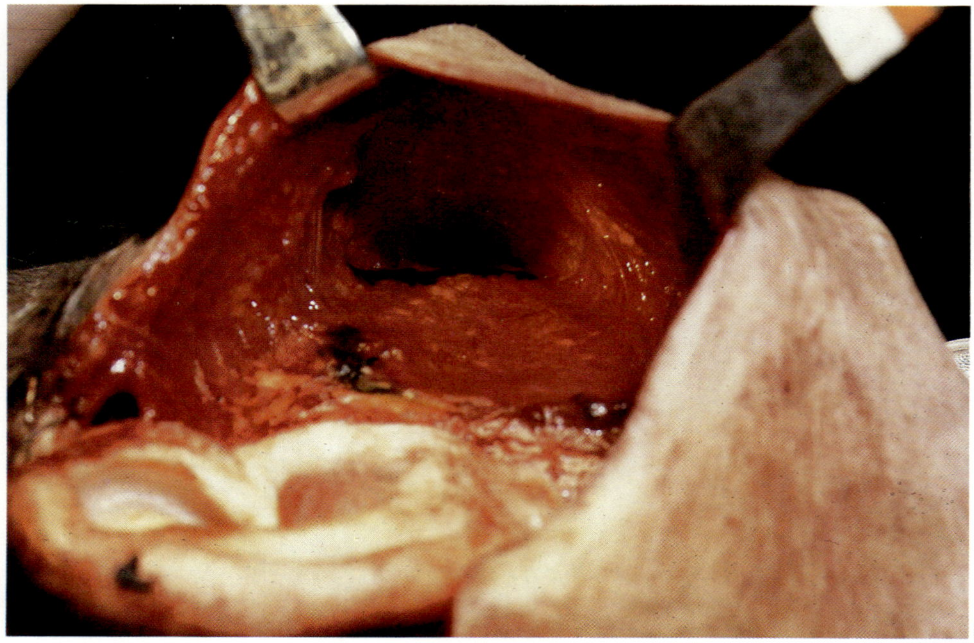

E

Figure 5–4 (continued)
E. Intraoperative (subcutaneous dissection medial to zygomaticus major muscle; epinephrine dilution 1:100,000).*

in a superior to inferior direction in the line of the zygomaticus major muscle, the dissection is safe. If the dissection is approached inferiorly and laterally to the zygomaticus major muscle, loss of a distinct plane may permit the scissors to slip under the zygomaticus major muscle and it is possible to injure some of the zygomatic branches of the facial nerve.

While there may be no single best approach to elevation of the SMAS, it is my belief that it is simpler to release the zygomatic nasolabial (upper) quadrilateral initially (before the buccal and mandibular quadrilaterals), as the adherent tissues in the two lower segments provide some stability when separating the firmly adherent areas of the zygomatic zone. If the zygomatic segment is released first, the adherent buccal and mandibular segments may, to some degree, hinder a complete release of the zygomatic segment. Therefore, after the buccal and mandibular segments are released, it may be necessary to release the nasolabial zone (zygomatic) segment further (medially) to achieve the results desired in the nasolabial fold.

Freeing the tissues to the nasolabial fold in this segment, particularly anterior (medial) to the zygomaticus major muscle is best accomplished by pressing the closed scissors toward the fold and spreading them in a vertical direction. As this is repeated, the areas separated can be joined by increasing the number of tunnels and ultimately joining them by transecting the remaining tissue bands.

Elevation of the Buccal Zone

The boundary of the buccal zone of the SMAS superiorly and inferiorly is the lower border of the zygomaticus major muscle and an imaginary horizontal line 1.0 to 1.5 cm below the buccal fat pad where the end fibers of the platysma muscle insert into the fibrous portion of the SMAS of the cheek, respectively. The posterior border is the line of entry to the sub-SMAS plane. Anteriorly the dissection extends to within 2.0 to 2.5 cm of the angle of the mouth (or until the desired results are achieved) (see Fig. 5–1). The quadrilateral (see Fig. 5–2) is broad posteriorly and narrows anteriorly, or just the reverse of the zygomatic (nasolabial fold) zone, which is broader anteriorly.

Along the posterior border of the buccal segment, the SMAS is easily separated from the deep fascia (see Fig. 5–2). This is accomplished by "tenting" or traction of the SMAS in a posterior and superior direction and with scissors, carefully and superficially transecting the tissue approximately 2 to 4 mm posterior to the fold of the tented SMAS. This technique of release accompanied by gentle spreading of the scissor blades in a horizontal (or vertical) direction maintains the level of dissection superficial to the deep fascia, which covers the branches of the facial nerve. To describe this in another fashion, release of the buccal segment is achieved by transecting the adherent plane in the dome of the SMAS (deep surface of the SMAS). As noted, the elevation in the area posterior (lateral) to the buccal fat pad is not difficult, as the layers of the plane are not tightly adherent.

Posterior to the region of the buccal fat pad, the SMAS and deep fascia become strongly adherent (see Fig. 5–2). The buccal branches of the facial nerve are visible, as the adherent fascial layers are quite thin. Also, the fascial plane between the SMAS and deep fascia is not well defined, and the proximity of the facial nerve branches contributes to make the dissection difficult and tedious. However, with patience and careful dissection, the anterior limit of the buccal quadrilateral, which, in essence, is the inferior continuation of the elevated nasolabial fold dissection (zygomatic zone dissection), can be established (Fig. 5–5).

The buccal fat pad is easily accessible, and although the results of its removal are difficult to evaluate, a portion can be removed in those patients in whom the cheeks are quite round or there are prominent pad-like folds extending from the angle of the mouth to the mandibular border. Coursing over the fat pad are the buccal branches of the facial nerve and small branches of the facial artery. The thin overlying fascia is penetrated by the closed scissor tips, or a mosquito clamp, and the fat pad teased free. The pad is clamped and transected, and the stump touched with the electrocautery.* The fat pad can be quite friable and at times may tear loose. When this occurs, moderately vigorous bleeding may result. If the stump retracts, it should be reintroduced to the surface and carefully inspected until the bleeding point is visualized. The electrocautery can then be utilized with accuracy, which protects the facial nerve from injury.

Elevation of the Mandibular Zone

The mandibular segment of the SMAS contains the extension of the platysma fibers over the mandible, the marginal mandibular branch of the facial nerve, and the cervical branch of the facial nerve.

*Bipolar electrocautery (see Chapter 3).

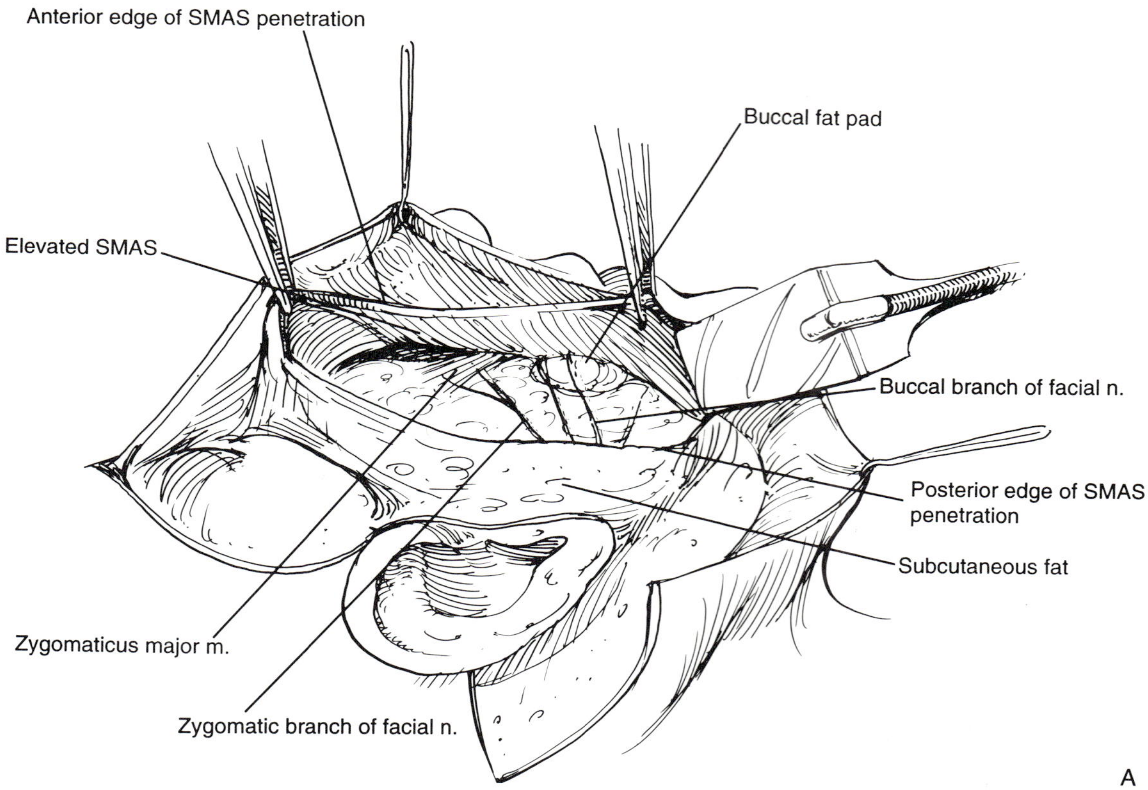

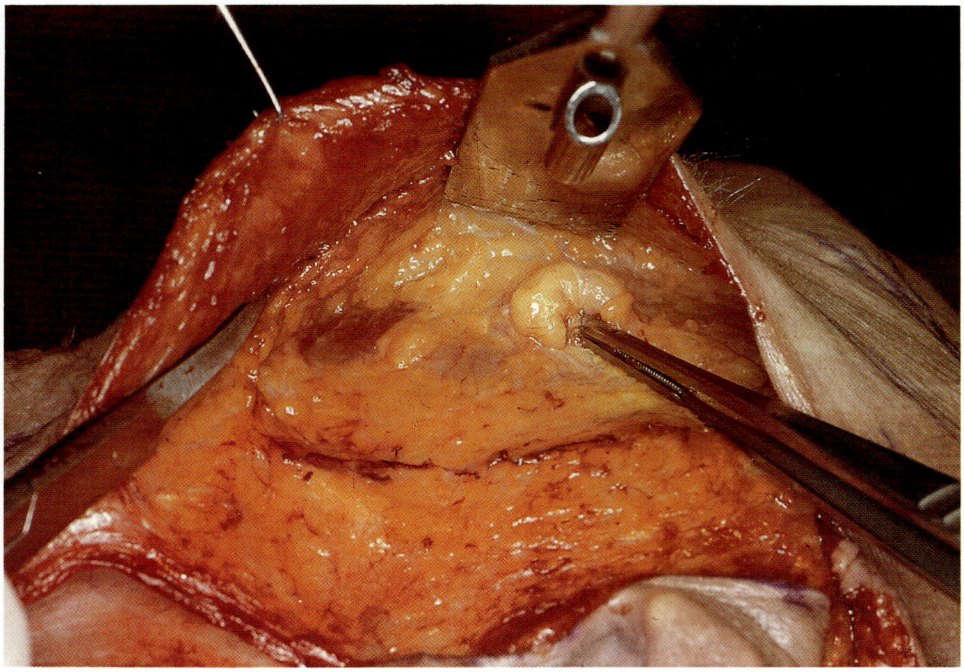

B

Figure 5–5. The buccal zone dissection: Release of the SMAS from the deep fascia of the head. **A.** Illustration of photograph (B) and (C). **B.** Cadaver.

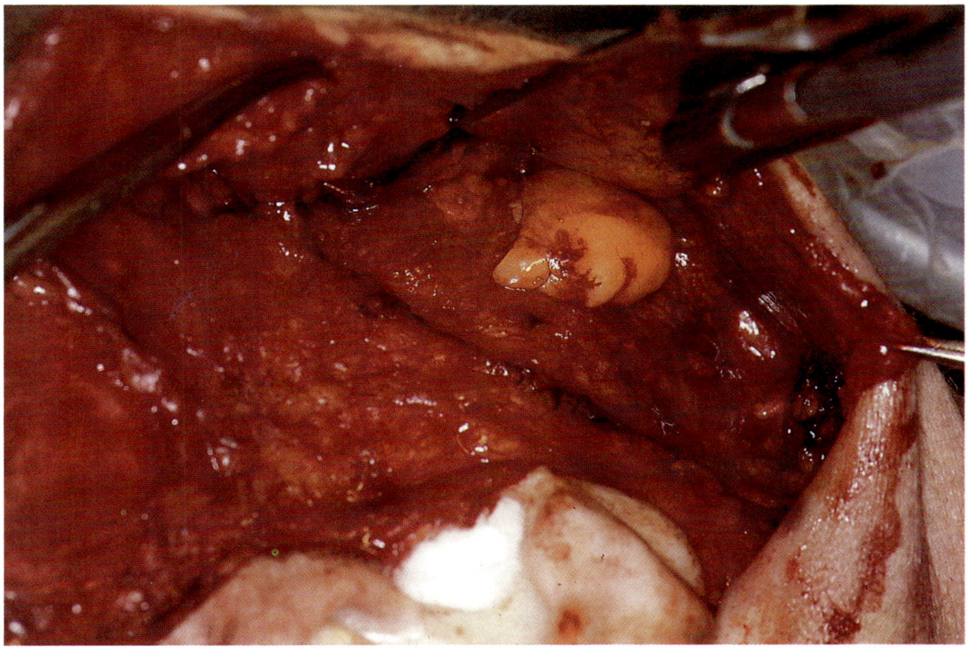

Figure 5–5 (continued) **C.** Intraoperative.

C

The boundaries of this segment (see Fig. 5–2) are the lateral border of the platysma muscle posteriorly, the integration of the platysma fibers with the fibrous tissue of the buccal segment of the SMAS superiorly (an imaginary horizontal line 1.0–1.5 cm inferior to the buccal fat pad), and an imaginary line approximately 2.5 to 3.0 cm caudad to the inferior border of the mandible inferiorly. The anterior border is a caudal extension of the anterior limit of the buccal segment, but with a moderate posterior curvilinear extension (see Fig. 5–1).

Effortless spreading of the scissors in a horizontal plane with the tips of the blades in the dome of the elevated SMAS, tightly against the platysma muscle, quickly frees the mandibular segment of the SMAS (Fig. 5–6). The deep fascia is well developed and the marginal mandibular branch of the facial nerve seldom seen.

As the marginal mandibular branch crosses the inferior border of the mandible anteriorly at the facial artery, it becomes superficial and remains superficial to the quadratus labii inferioris and the mentalis muscles in its supply (in contrast to the superficial muscles of the face in which the supply enters the deep surface of the muscle). Damage to this branch causes paresis of the nerve supply and loss of depressor action of the lower lip.

The cervical branch of the facial nerve can be preserved because the submandibular elevation of the platysma muscle does not have to be extensive to provide adequate advancement of the SMAS platysma of the cheek. When a more extensive subplatysma dissection and/or transection of a portion of the muscle is done, loss of depressor function of the lower lip in a sub-SMAS facelift is usually a result of damage to the platysma muscle, and is considered a pseudomandibular branch paresis[2] as recovery is almost always complete.

Figure 5–6. The mandibular zone dissection: Release of the SMAS from the deep fascia of the head. **A.** Illustration of photograph (B) and (C). **B.** Cadaver.

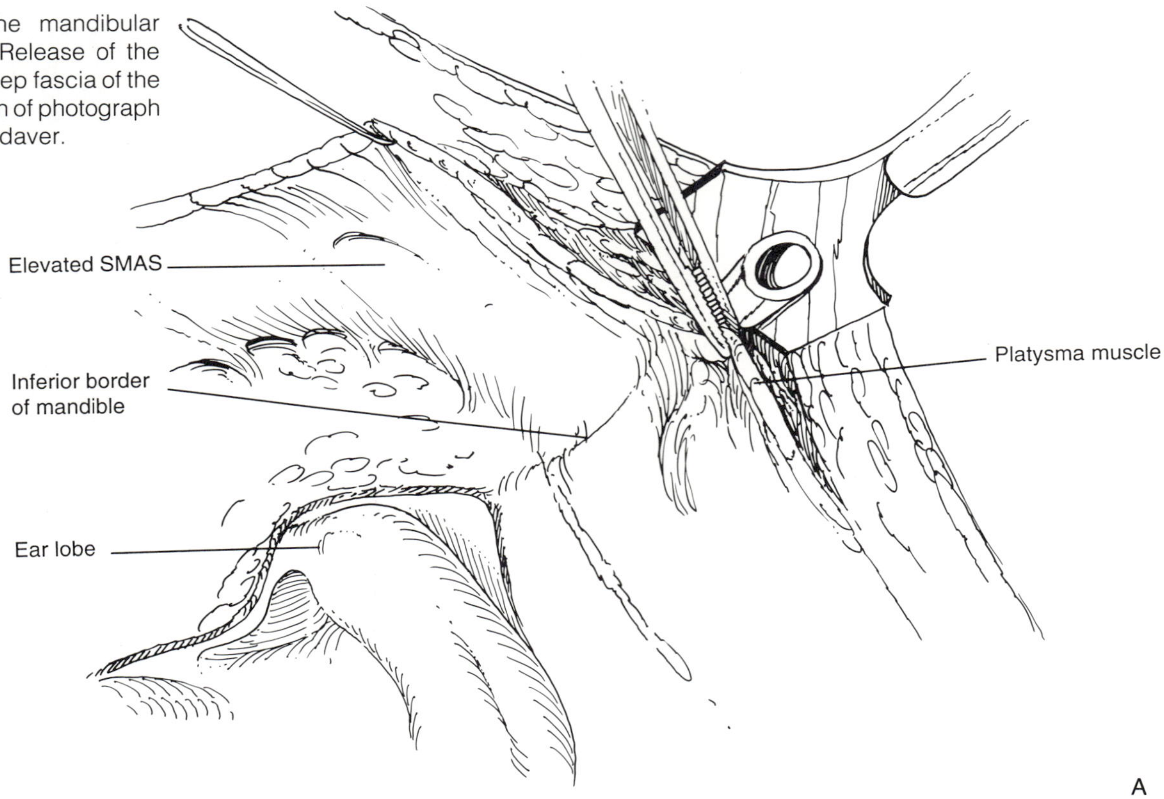

A

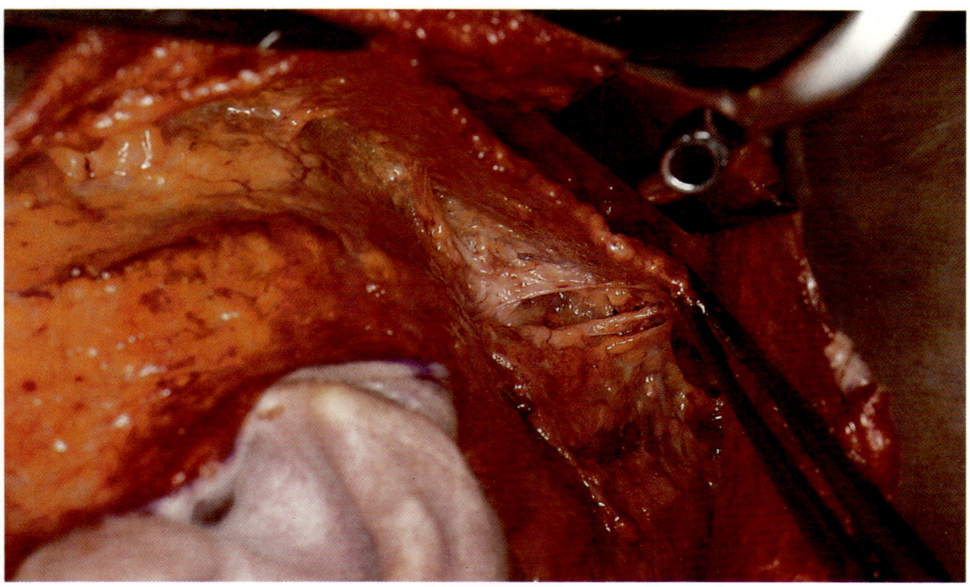

B

Figure 5–6 (continued) C. Intraoperative.

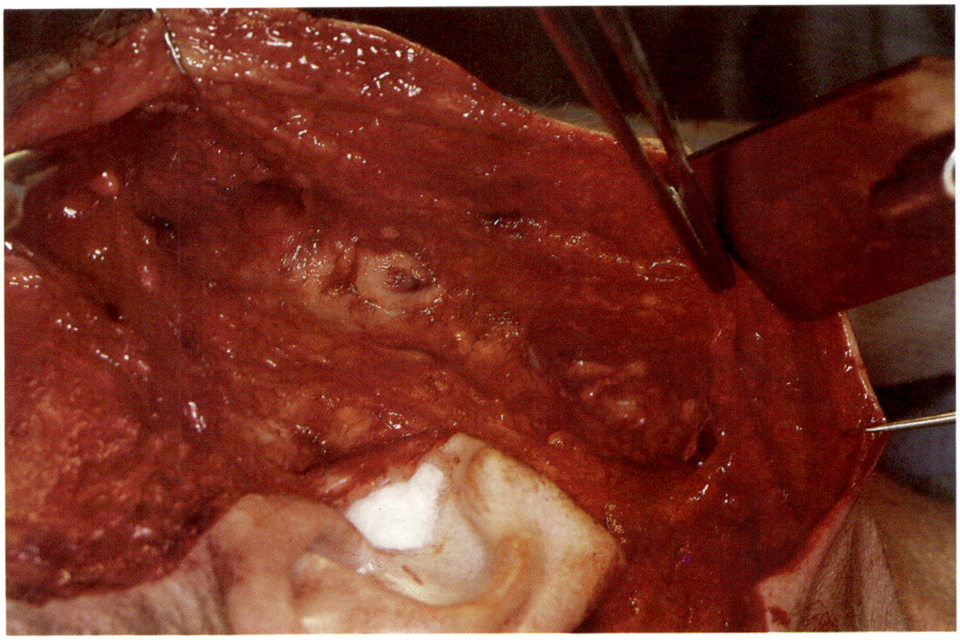

C

Cephalad and Posterior Advancement of SMAS–Platysma Muscle

The repair of the anatomical changes of aging requires that the involved tissues be released widely to provide the freedom to advance the tissues to a new location ("new bed"), thereby correcting the defect without undue tension. It is unusual to expect a satisfactory and long-lasting repair of tissue defects by forceful "pulling" or advancement of tissues when there is constant, forceful, residual countertraction that results from an inadequate release of the tissues. The extent of the release of the SMAS meets the criterion of this surgical principle.

The extent of the elevation of the SMAS medially, superiorly, and inferiorly (zygomatic, buccal, and mandibular zones) (Fig. 5–7) illustrates the magnitude of the release of the SMAS necessary to provide the restoration of the attenuated tissues of the face.

The posterior border of the SMAS (Fig. 5–8) is grasped, elevated, and advanced posterosuperiorly toward the ear by the inferior clamp and more cephalad and posteriorly by the upper clamp to its new location on the deep fascia. With an extensive release of the SMAS, the platysma muscle at the caudad extension of the SMAS-platysma elevation may restrict its posterosuperior advancement. To achieve the maximum advancement of the SMAS-platysma muscle, the posterior border of the platysma muscle is partially transected (Fig. 5–9) to the extent necessary to permit full cephalad-posterior advancement of the mandibular segment. The line of transection of the posterior border of the platysma muscle is placed in an oblique inferior direction and extends only as far as necessary to relieve any tension (countertraction) on the advanced SMAS. This releases the SMAS–platysma muscle of the cheek (which has been elevated from the deep fascia) from the platysma

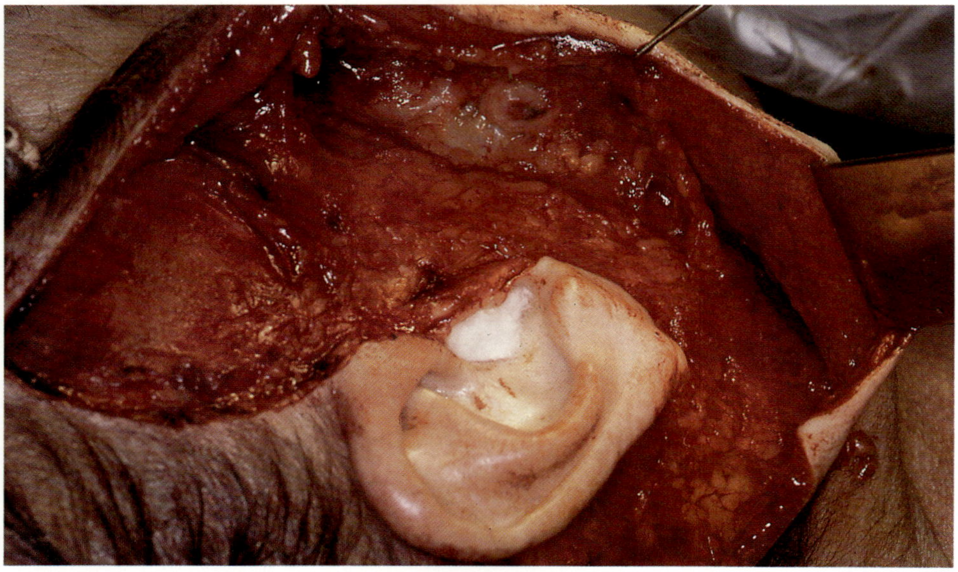

Figure 5–7. The extent of the elevation of the SMAS: Zygomatic, buccal, and mandibular zones.

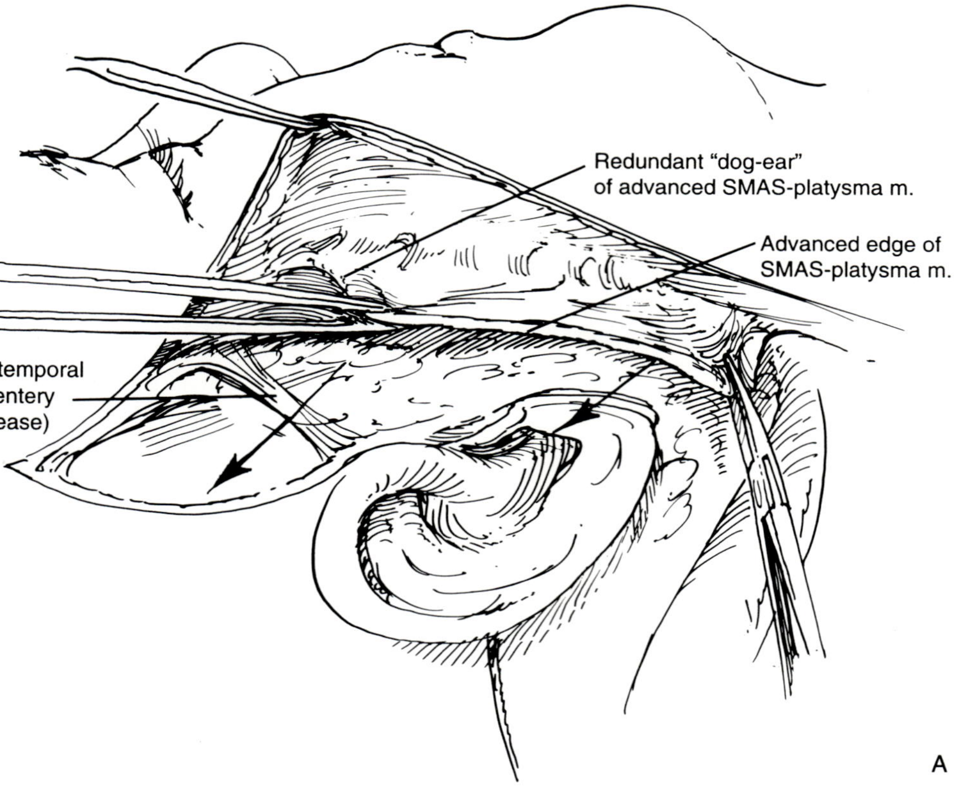

Figure 5–8. Advancement of the complex morphological unit (skin, subcutaneous fat, and SMAS) of the face and neck. **A.** Illustration of photograph (B).

Figure 5–8 (continued) **B.** Cadaver.

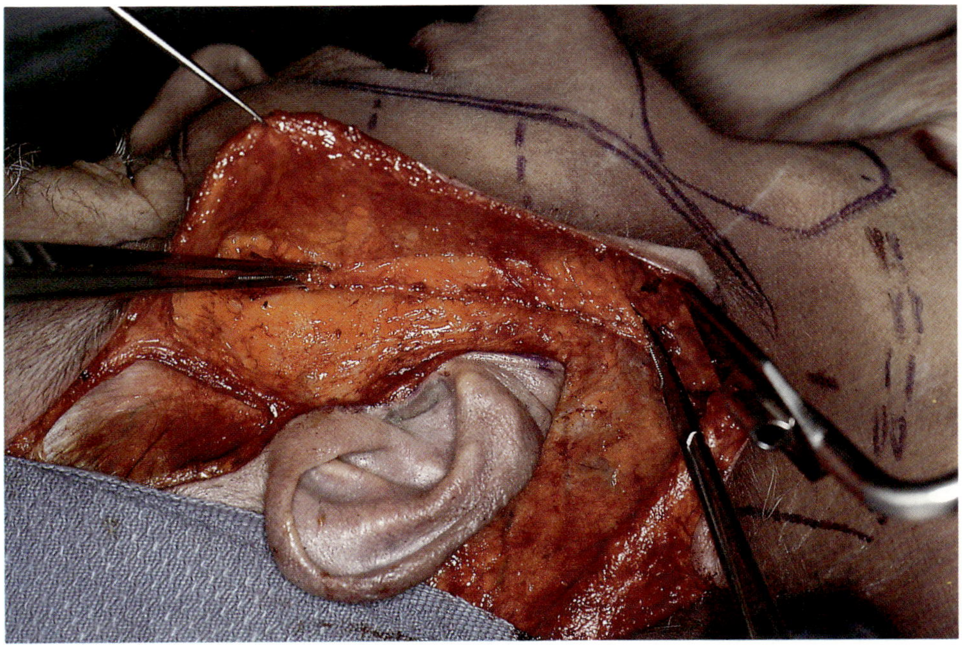

B

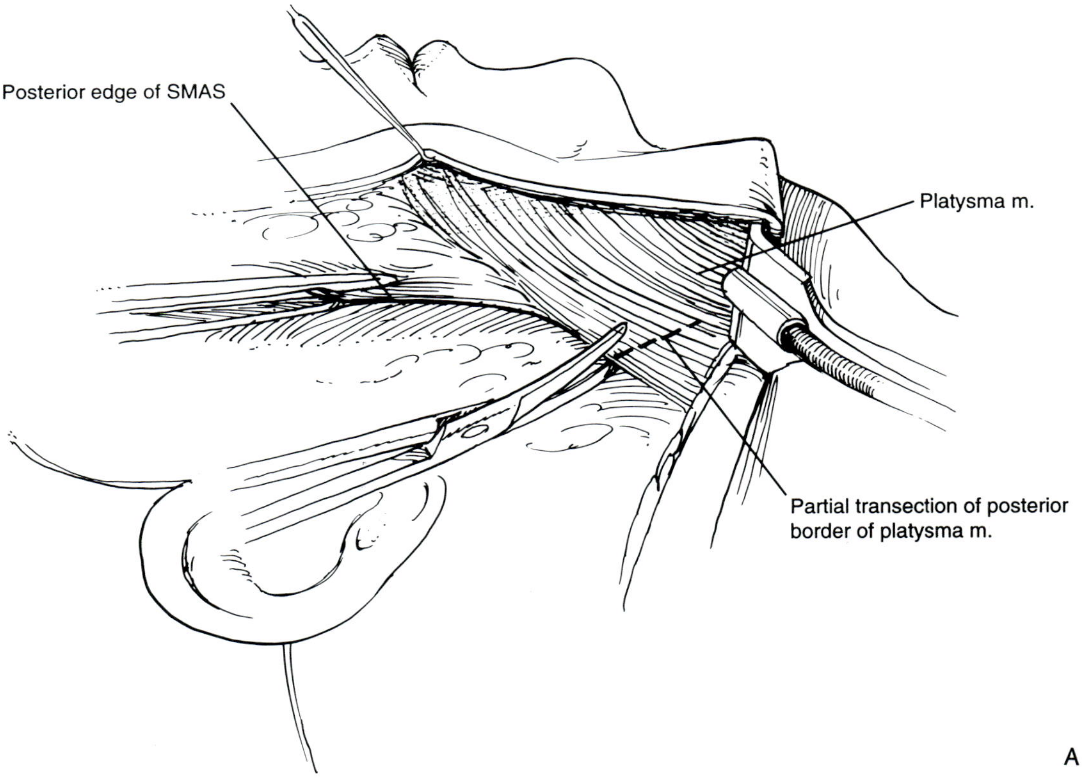

A

Figure 5–9. Release of the SMAS–platysma muscle of the face from the platysma muscle of the neck: Transection of the posterior border of the platysma muscle. **A.** Illustration of photograph (B).

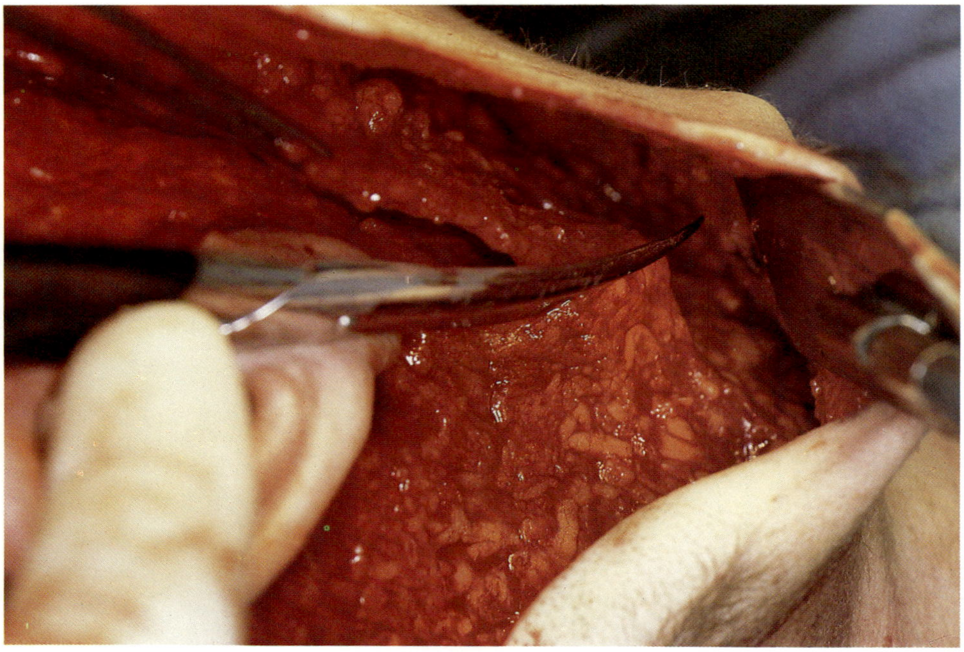

B

Figure 5–9 (continued) B. Intraoperative.

muscle of the neck (which remains adherent to the deep fascia below the transection). It should be emphasized that transection of the posterior border of the platysma muscle should be restricted. Partial transection of the posterior border of the platysma muscle adds little to the cervicomandibular contours, and may damage some of the cervical branches of the facial nerve to the platysma muscle.

With cephalad-posterior advancement of the SMAS, a "dog-ear" may form at its superior aspect[3] (Figs. 5–8 to 5–10). The posterior border of the SMAS in this region is transected medially at the most cephalad point of its advancement (see Fig. 5–10A). The advanced SMAS overlapping the incision is excised (see Fig. 5–10B). Only the amount of the "dog-ear" necessary to provide a smooth contour is excised. If desired, the redundant portion of the SMAS may be left and with advancement and closure of the SMAS provides some minimal increase in tissue fullness to the malar area. More often than not, the release of the lower portion of the orbicularis oculi and the subcutaneous dissection medially provide sufficient release of the tissues so that the advancement of the SMAS does not create any "dog-ear" of the SMAS, or is so insignificant it requires no excision.

Closure of the Advanced SMAS and Resection of the Redundant SMAS

The advanced SMAS is approximated with the posterior segment of the superficial fascia of the preauricular region from cephalad to caudad beginning at the malar prominence/zygoma level. The malar suture is the first and most important suture in the closure of the SMAS. It determines the tension necessary for the SMAS closure and in turn adjusts the nasolabial fold.

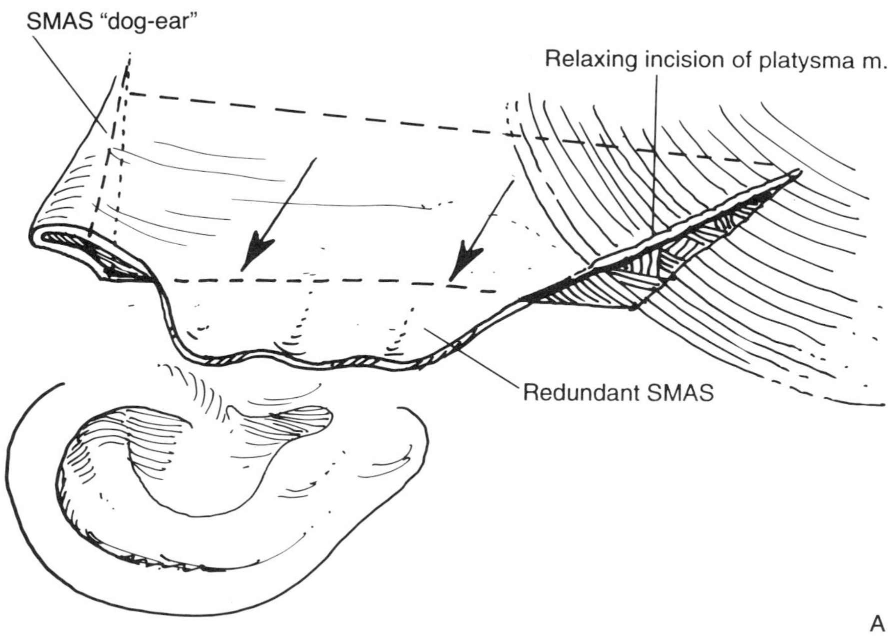

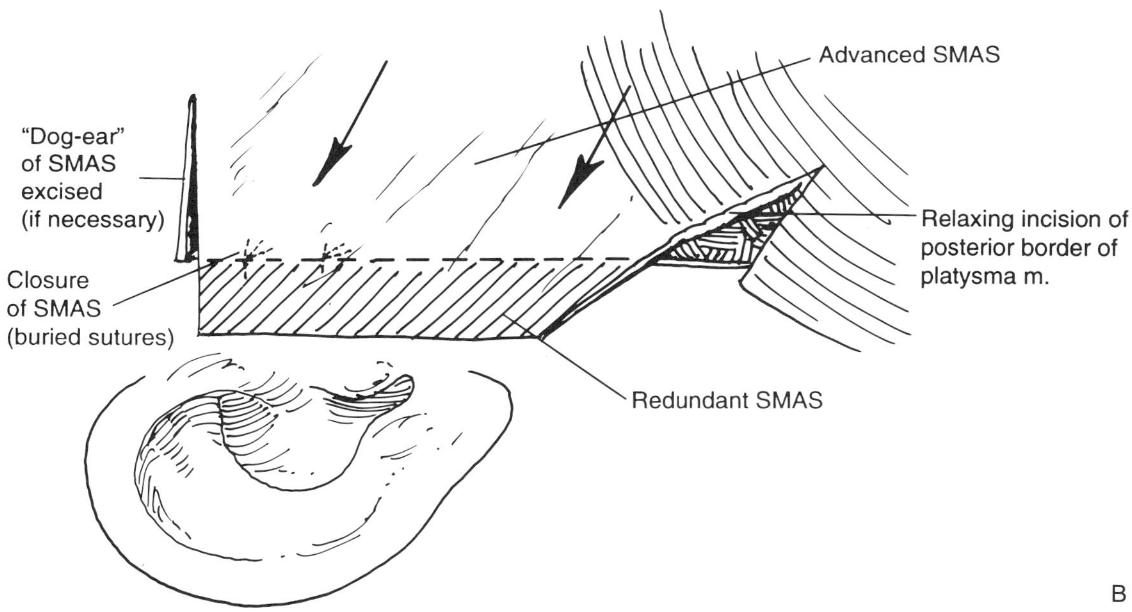

Figure 5–10. Superior and posterior advancement of the SMAS. **A.** Possible cephalad "dog-ear" of SMAS. **B.** Excision of a "dog-ear" from the SMAS advancement. Redundant SMAS overlaps subcutaneous dissection of the preauricular area.

Fig. 5–11B, C shows the posterior border of the elevated SMAS. The location of the initial suture (3–0 Vicryl, no. 683 Ethicon) on the deep surface of the SMAS demonstrates the placement, or distance of the advancement of the SMAS, possible with the first or malar/zygoma suture. Fig. 5–11D, E indicates the amount of tension of the closure of the advanced SMAS, where the deep surface of the advanced SMAS approximates the posterior edge of the area of penetration of the SMAS in the region of the zygoma/malar prominence.

To determine the amount of tension on the closure, the elevated SMAS (complex morphologic unit) is grasped with mosquito clamps at its cephalad and caudad extent, and these are held by an assistant. A suture (3–0 Vicryl, no. 683 Ethicon) is placed through the deep fascia of the malar prominence or zygoma, also incorporating the posterior edge of the superficial fascia (Fig. 5–11). The posterior edge of the line of penetration of the superficial fascia is grasped with Brown-Adson forceps and pushed anteriorly (medially) to eliminate slack in the tissues. The mosquito clamps on the posterior edge of the elevated SMAS are pulled posteriorly (laterally) to overlap the tips of the Brown-Adson. The overlap of the SMAS can range from 2.0 to 3.5 cm. Approximately one centimeter anterior to the line where the undersurface of the SMAS (deep) and the advanced posterior segment of the superficial fascia overlap (tips of the Brown-Adson thumb forceps) and slightly caudad to the level of the suture in the posterior segment of the SMAS, the suture of the malar region is introduced into the deep surface of the SMAS (Fig. 5–11). The suture is snugged down and the results observed. If it is not satisfactory (too much or too little tension), another trial placement is done. If the tension is considered satisfactory and the correction of the nasolabial fold is sufficient, the suture is tied. The balance of the closure of the advanced SMAS and the posterior segment of the superficial fascia is accomplished in the same manner.

The tension of the advancement of the SMAS, particularly in the buccal segment, can be overdone, which with healing creates a taut line of the cheek in the submalar region (caudad) between the ear and the corner of the mouth. This is most noticeable on animation and unfortunately, it may not resolve completely with the passage of time.

The advancement and closure of the SMAS results in the anterior portion of the SMAS overlapping the posterior SMAS in the preauricular region. The overlapped, redundant SMAS is excised (Fig. 5–12). If the overlapped portion of the SMAS is thin, it does not have to be trimmed. Utilization of the excess SMAS in various ways to add further support to the SMAS closure does not seem to be of any great additional value.

The dissection and repair are complete (Fig. 5–13), and the skin redraping and closure can commence.

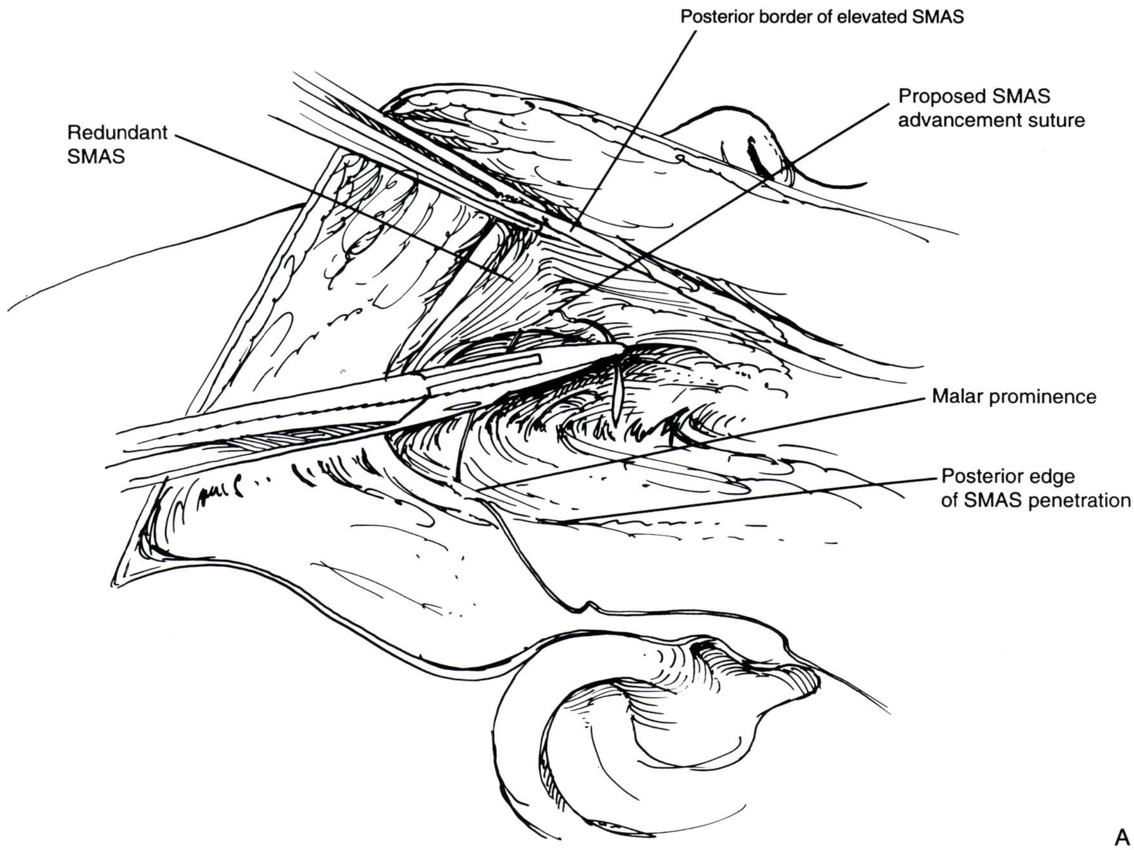

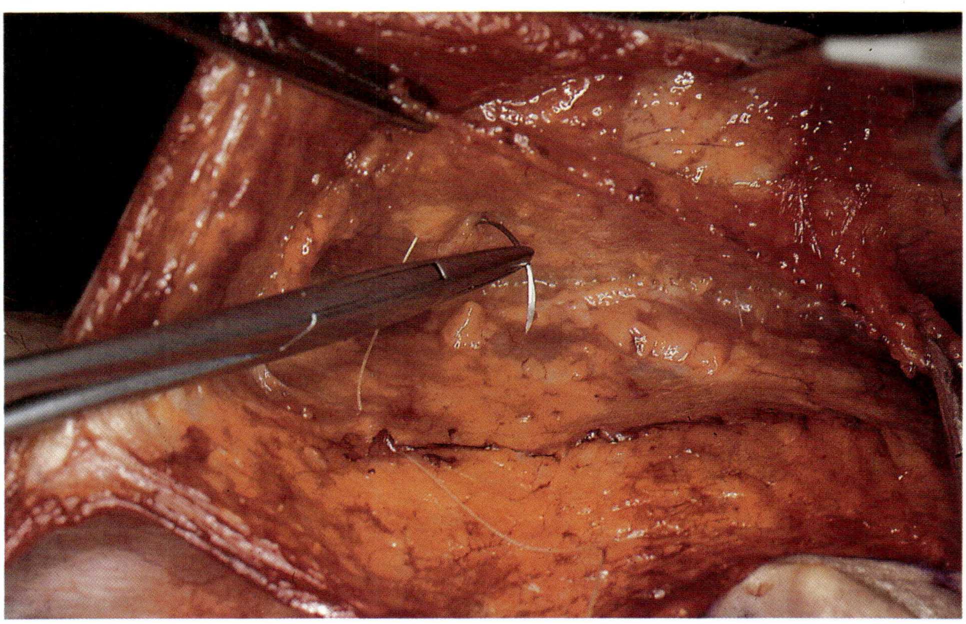

Figure 5–11. The initial suture and closure of the advanced SMAS. **A.** Illustration of photograph (B) and (C). **B.** Cadaver.

Figure 5–11 (continued) **C.** Intraoperative. **D.** Cadaver.

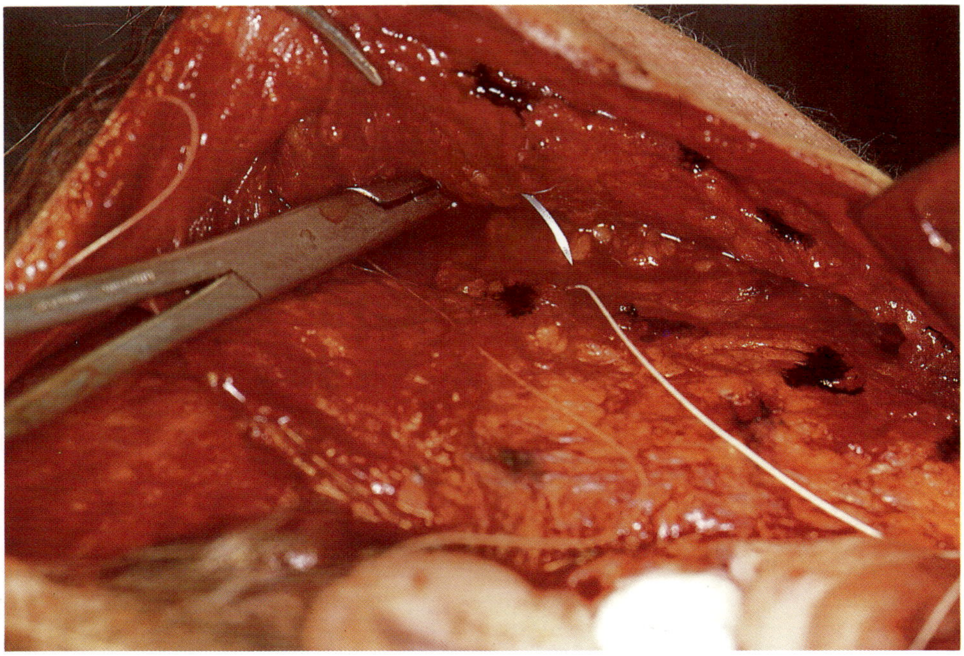

C

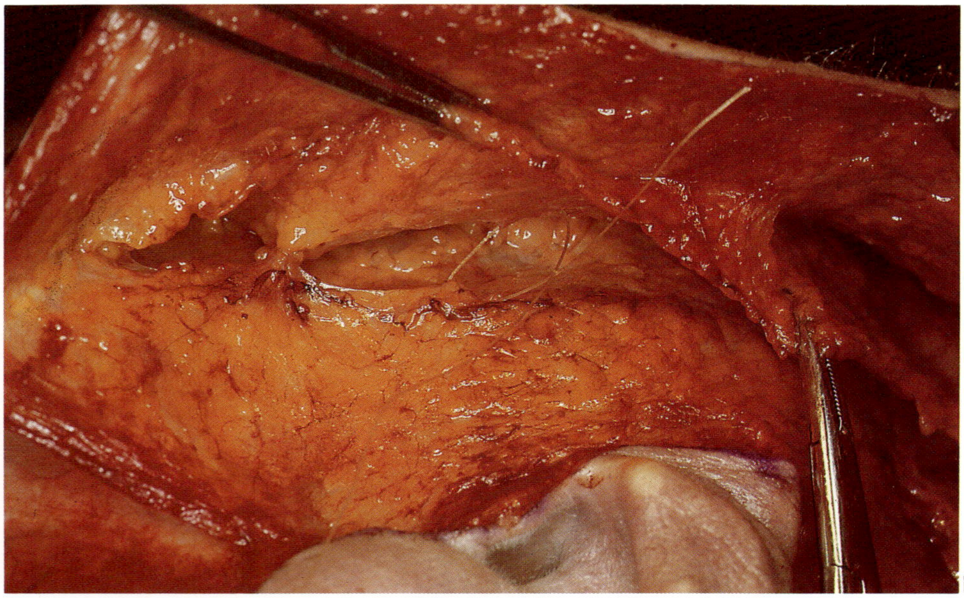

D

Figure 5–11 (continued) **E.** Intraoperative.

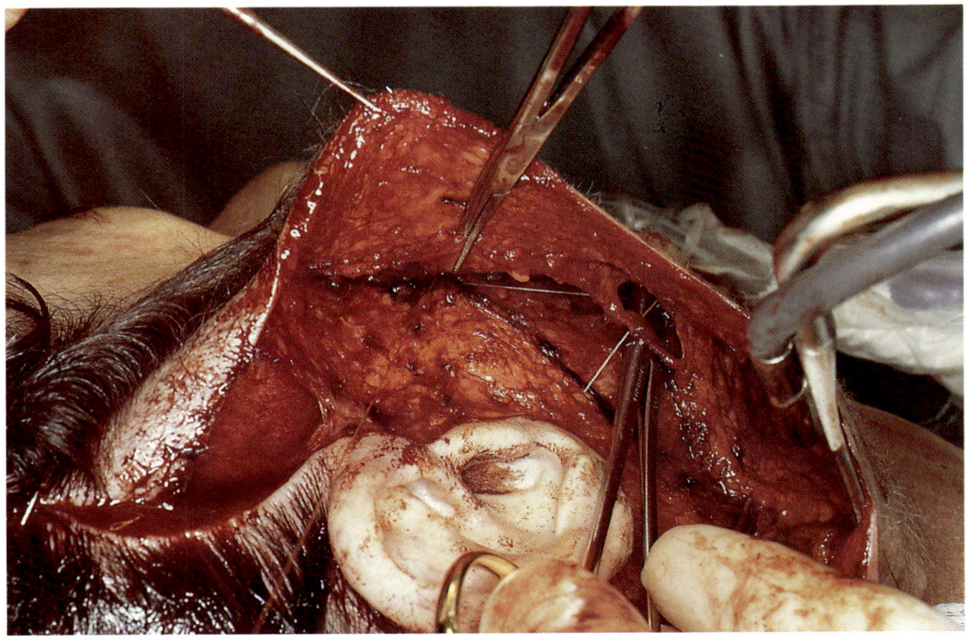

E

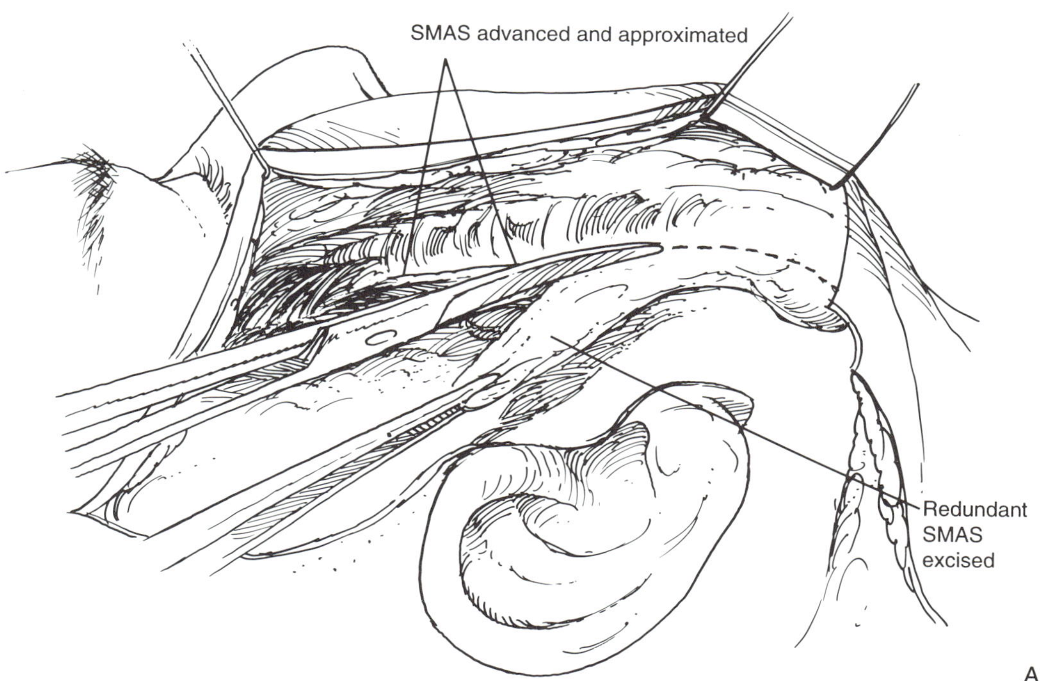

A

Figure 5–12. The excision of the redundant SMAS of the preauricular area. **A.** Illustration of photograph (B).

Figure 5–12 (continued) **B.** Cadaver. **C.** Intraoperative.

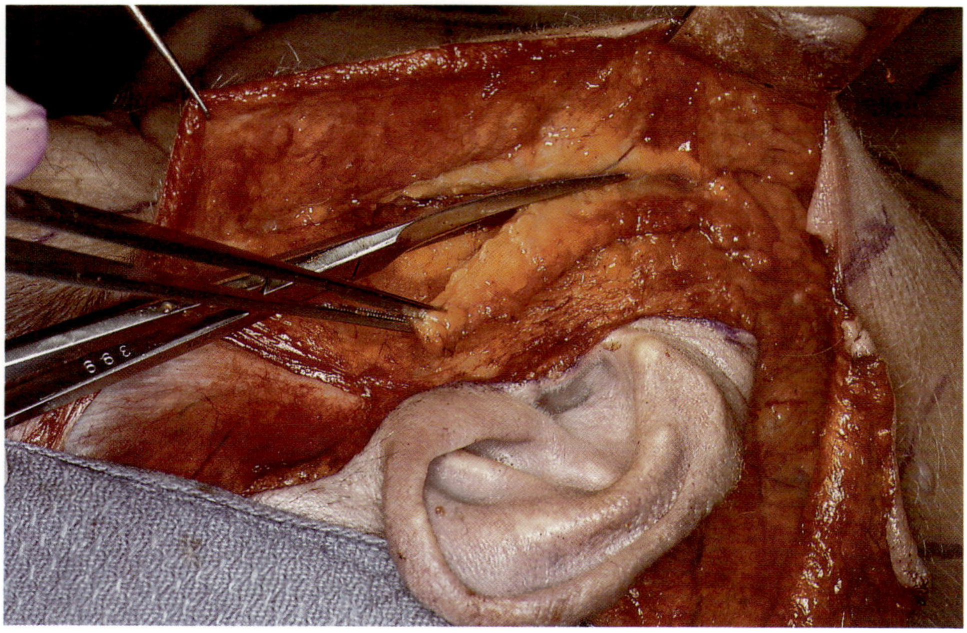

B

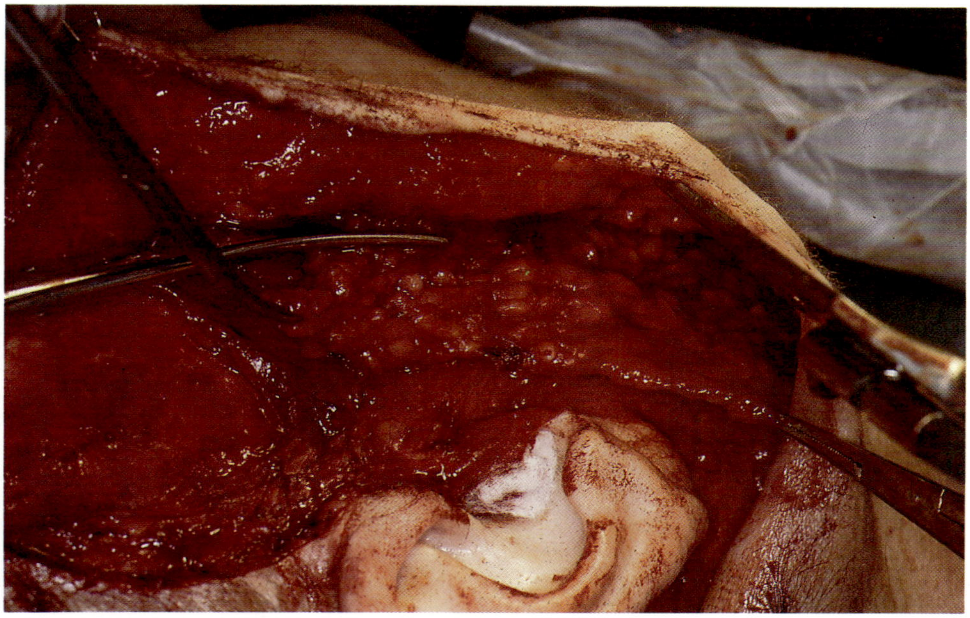

C

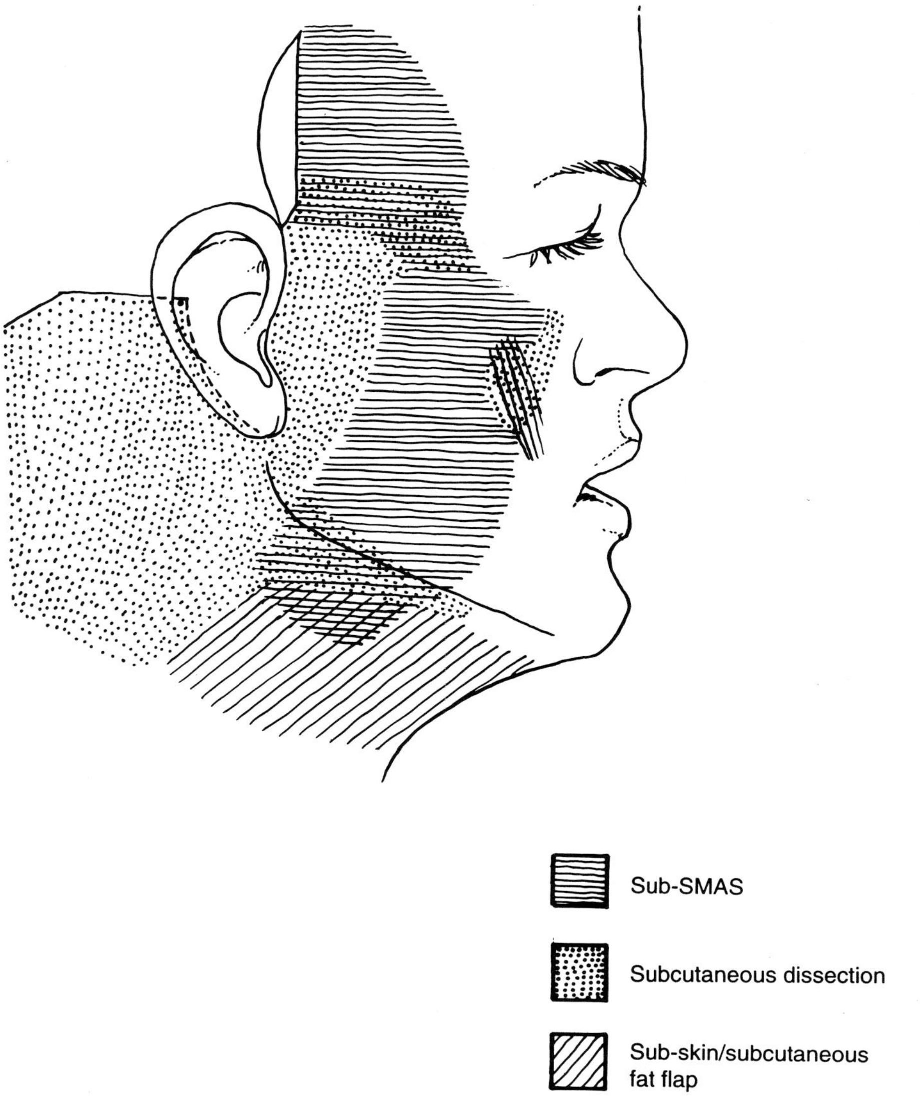

Figure 5–13. The area and level of the complete dissection of the face and neck.

References

1. Skoog, T.: Plastic Surgery—New Methods, Philadelphia, W.B. Saunders, 1974, p. 313.
2. Ellenbogen, R.: Pseudoparalysis of the mandibular branch of the facial nerve after platysmal face-lift operation. Plast. Reconstr. Surg. 1979; 63:364–368.
3. Owsley, J.Q.: Platysma-facial rhytidectomy. Plast. Reconstr. Surg. 1977; 60: 843–850.

SIX

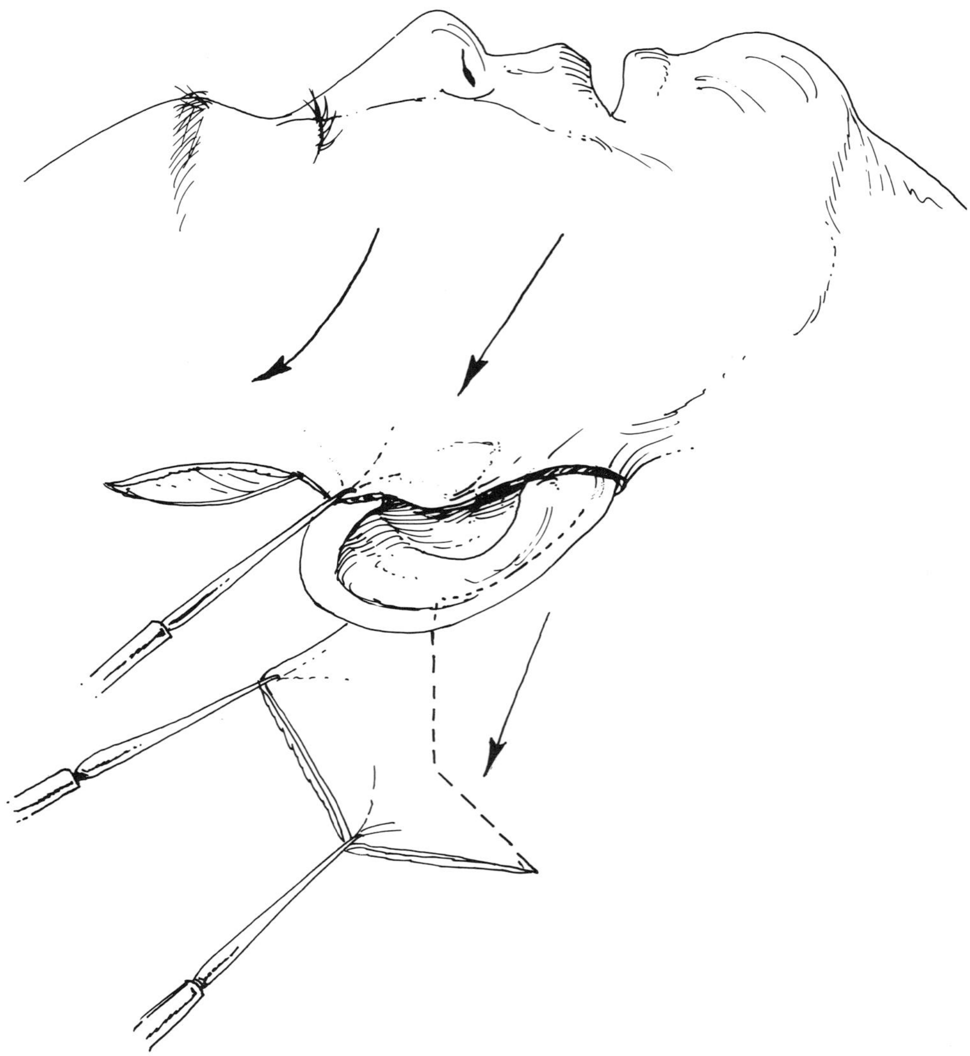

The Redrape and Excision/Closure of the Skin of the Face and Cervical Region

The skin closure, while not technically difficult when done correctly, produces minimal scarring (in most cases). Good scars bring many significant and repetitive compliments from close observers and reinforces the results in the patient's mind.

The important elements of the skin closure are:

1. The position and direction of the redrape of the preauricular and postauricular skin
2. The tension to be placed on the skin flaps
3. The placement of the temporal and postauricular skin flap sutures
4. The management of the redundant skin at the posterior extent of the occipital incision
5. The trimming of the skin around the ear
6. Obtaining a satisfactory appearance of the tragus in a tragal rim closure

Table 6–1 outlines the intraoperative sequence of the skin redrape and wound closure.

Bidirectional Vectors of the Skin: Redraping of the Cheek and Cervical Skin Flaps

The objective of the redraping of the excess skin of the face from aging is to remove the maximum amount possible, to provide a smooth skin redraping of the face and neck contours and to minimize the amount of scarring from the closure. Additionally the hairline should be restored as closely as possible to normal. The key steps in this process are a bidirectional redrape of the skin

Table 6–1. The Intraoperative Sequence of the Skin Redrape and Wound Closure

1.	Redrape of preauricular and postauricular skin
2.	Placement of the temporal suture
3.	Trimming and closure of the temporal wound
4.	Placement of the postauricular suture
5.	Trimming of the occipital skin
6.	Closure of the occipital wound
7.	Trimming of the postauricular skin
8.	Trimming of the preauricular skin
9.	Trimming of the tragus skin insert
10.	Closure of the preauricular and postauricular wound

of the face and neck and the setting of the redraping in the proper position by placement of the temporal and postauricular sutures.

The skin of the cheek is pulled superiorly and posteriorly, and the cervical flap of the postauricular region is directed more posteriorly than the preauricular flap, but also superiorly depending on the characteristics of the skin and the extent of the aging changes. The pivot point of the divergence of the direction of the vectors is the earlobe. While the direction of the advancement of skin is extremely variable, depending on the characteristics of the skin and the extent of the aging changes in general, the direction of the advancement of the skin of the cheek approximates the direction of the vectors shown in Fig. 6–1. The cheek skin is advanced almost equally superiorly and posteriorly, whereas the occipital–posterior cervical flap is advanced superiorly and rotated posteriorly. Stated another way, the occipital–posterior cervical flap is advanced along a line parallel to the postauricular sulcus, with the postauricular skin edge of the occipital–posterior cervical flap touching or minimally overlapping the postauricular skin edge on the medial (posterior) surface of the ear.

To prevent large "dog-ears" at the end of the occipital incision, there is a tendency to advance the postauricular flap in a more vertical direction, or anteriorly toward the posterior surface of the ear. This combined with the posterior advancement of the cheek skin can cause bunching of the skin below the earlobe. In faces with considerable amounts of redundant skin and severe wrinkling, the "dog-ear" in the posterior occipital region may be sizable; however, the caudad angling of the horizontal occipital incision allows this increased posterior rotation of the posterior cervical skin flap, which permits easy removal of the excess tissue. While this may create a step deformity of the hairline behind the ear, this is much preferable to a bunching of skin visible below the earlobe.

Frequently the posterior cervical flap may require further release along its posterior aspect to ensure a smooth drape of the region. Absent this release, the flap may have visible permanent vertical folds in the region, particularly in patients with large amounts of excess skin and extreme solar radiation damage.

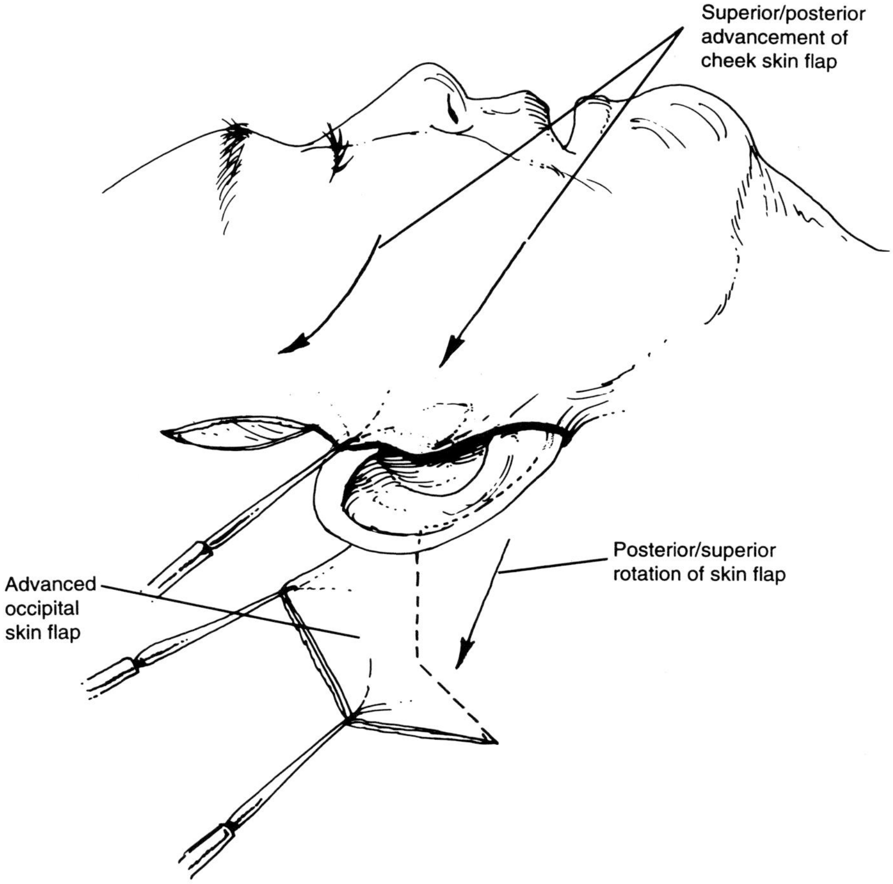

Figure 6–1. Bidirectional advancement of the cheek and postauricular skin flaps.

Placement of the Temporal Suture

Once the skin is redraped and the direction of the preauricular and postauricular flaps are determined, the temporal suture (3–0 plain catgut, no. 822, Ethicon) is placed (Fig. 6–2A).* Because the advanced SMAS-platysma muscle-skin subcutaneous tissue complex (compound morphologic unit) is intact in the cheek, the subdermal skin elevation in the preauricular region covers the lower portion of the ear without tension and remains in a posterior-superior position. With a skin hook in the cheek flap and forceps (Brown-Adson) on the posterior skin edge of the temporal incision, opposing traction is placed on the skin flaps and the posterior element of the temporal incision just above the junction of the helix of the ear and the skull (see Fig. 6–2B). The direction of the traction at the level of the junction of the helix of the ear and the skull is mainly horizontal (posterior) because of the redraped skin (superior/posterior) and the repair of the intact SMAS-platysma-skin complex have advanced the tissues to the desired level.

*The core set of instruments specified in Chapter 3 are employed.

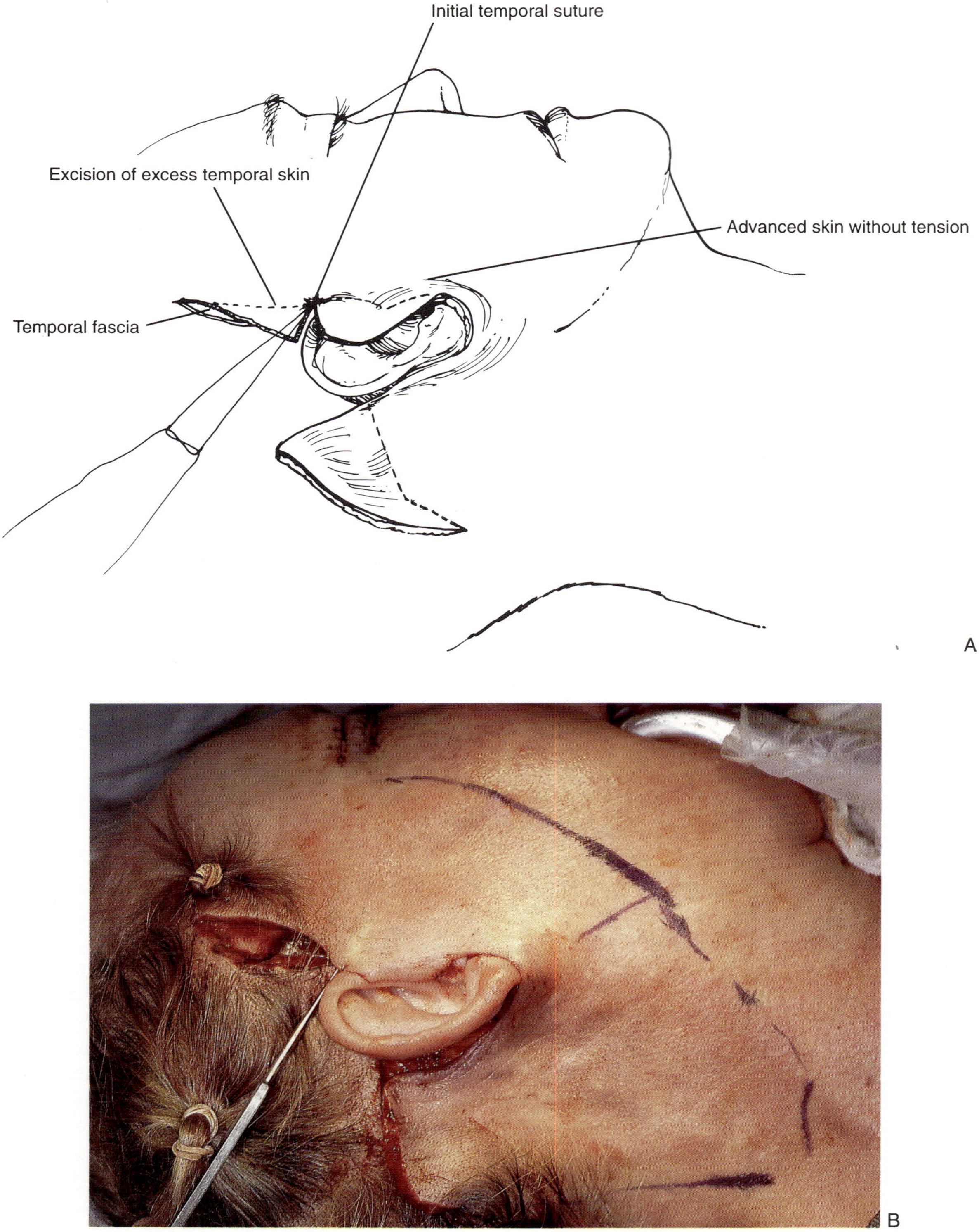

Figure 6–2. The placement of the initial temporal suture. **A.** Illustration of photograph (B). **B.** Intraoperative.

The skin flap is incised to a point (see Fig. 6–2A) estimated to provide a moderate amount of tension. This suture (3–0 plain catgut, no. 822, Ethicon) sets the tension of the temporal advancement. The redundant scalp is trimmed. After trimming, the remainder of the temporal wound is closed with 3–0 plain catgut suture (no. 822, Ethicon) (or the operator's choice of closure). While the temporal suture may be under moderate tension, the trim of any redundant scalp in this region should cause only minimal tension on the temporal closure. Too much tension on the temporal scalp closure may cause temporary or permanent hair loss.

The superficial temporal fascia mesentery created by the elevation of the superficial temporal fascia and the subdermal elevation of the skin lateral to the orbit which overlaps the lower portion of the elevated superficial temporal fascia may restrict the cephalad (superior) and lateral (posterior) advancement of the redraping of the scalp in the temporal area. When this occurs the base of the mesentery is transected at its lateral attachment (posterior) sufficiently to permit a smooth redraping of the skin lateral (posterior) to the orbit. This is accomplished by sharp dissection at the base of the mesentery laterally, but after the initial release is established, blunt dissection can be employed. Usually, only minimal release is necessary, but to protect the frontal branch of the facial nerve the maximum limit of the release should be only about half the mesentery's width. If this does not permit a smooth redrape of the skin lateral to the orbit, the subdermal elevation of the skin should be extended cephalad to overlap more of the elevated superficial temporal fascia.

If the amount of relaxed skin of the cheek is large, the advancement of the skin of the cheek may raise the hairline (sideburn) higher than desired. When this occurs, a horizontal wedge of skin below the sideburn may be removed and the hair-bearing area advanced in a caudad direction or at least retained at a lower level. To some degree, this minimizes an extreme elevation of the hairline and an otherwise obvious lack of a normal hairline.

Placement of the Postauricular Suture

After the temporal closure is complete, the ear is folded anteriorly, being certain this includes the lower portion of the ear and the earlobe covered by the excess skin (Fig. 6–3A, B). The wound edge of the posterior cervical flap lies opposite the ear wound edge and is not pulled anteriorly because the directional drape (arrow) of the skin is, as mentioned (see Fig. 6–1), more posterior, or at a greater angle from the vertical on the head than that of the cheek advancement. In effect, the postauricular skin edge of the occipital–posterior cervical flap is advanced cephalad and adjacent to the skin edge of the postauricular incision on the ear. (When the anterior traction on the ear is released, there should be very little posterior auricular skin to trim.) With the skin flap in this position and under moderate tension and the ear held in the anterior position, the wound edge is incised sufficiently to place an interrupted 3–0 plain catgut (no. 822, Ethicon) suture (see Fig. 6–3A).

The suture is placed in the skin edge below the incision of the posterior cervical flap, passes through the fascia of the mastoid region for anchorage, and emerges from the skin at the angle created by the limbs of the postauric-

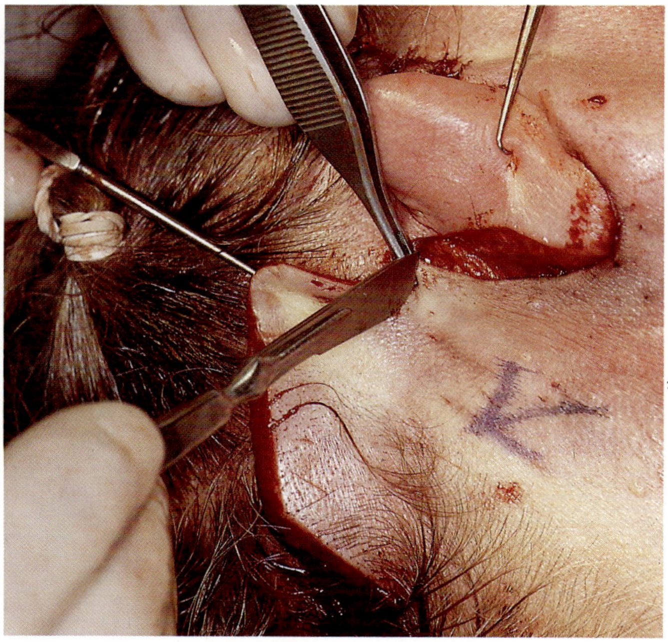

A

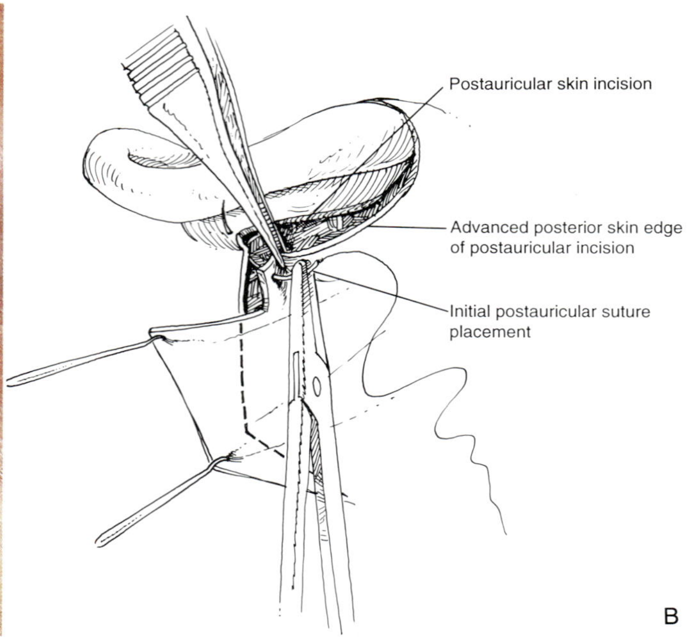

B

Figure 6–3. The placement of the initial postauricular suture. **A.** Incision of the advanced posterior cervical skin flap. **B.** Illustration of photograph (C). **C.** Suture placement, intraoperative.

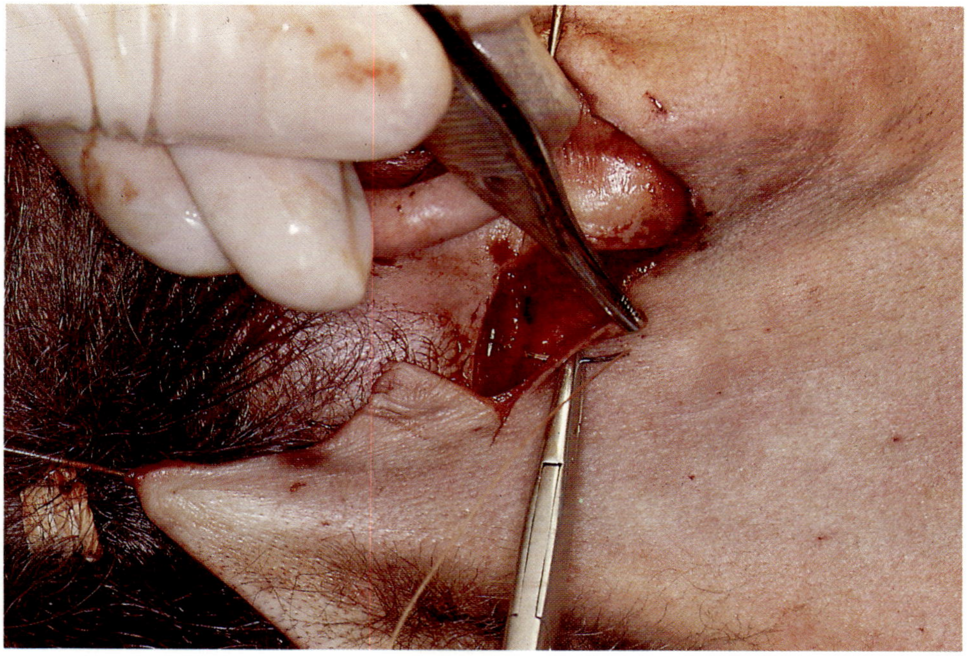

C

ular and occipital incisions (see Fig. 6–3B). The temporal and postauricular sutures (see Fig. 6–2A; Fig. 6–4B) maintain the bidirectional redraping of the cheek and the occipital posterior cervical flap, while the remaining skin is trimmed and the wound closed.

Trimming of the Occipital Skin Flap Redundancy

Traction in the direction of the angle of the postauricular flap redrape (see Fig. 6–1) is applied to the posterior cervical skin flap. A point on the skin flap at the angle of the caudad extension of the occipital incision (see Fig. 6–4) is grasped and traction applied. The skin flap is incised to the point of the angle on the cephalad edge of the occipital incision (see Fig. 6–4). The scalp posterior to this incision is excised and the portion of the caudad angulation of the occipital incision immediately closed with interrupted 3–0 plain catgut (no. 822, Ethicon).

The area in the scalp at the posterior end of the occipital limb closure at times may be slightly bunched and form a small knob; however, it is usually not of consequence and further "chasing" of it may not totally correct it. At a future date, this can be removed, though it is rarely necessary.

The closure of the posterior limb of the occipital wound and the postauricular suture are support points for the occipital flap and reduce the tension on the horizontal limb of the occipital wound closure.

The remaining skin on the occipital flap represents a quadrilateral of redundant tissue (Fig. 6–5). Sufficient traction is applied to this flap so that after excision of the redundancy, the skin edges are separated by about 1 cm (Fig. 6–6). The posterior cervical flap is lying in its advanced position under minimal to moderate tension and is held by the angled or oblique limb of the posterior extent of the occipital incision and the postauricular suture at the anterior end. The horizontal limb of the occipital incision is closed with a continuous dermal suture of 3–0 plain catgut (no. 822, Ethicon). (A dermal suture closure reduces scarring sometimes seen with interrupted sutures or staples.)

Approximating the skin edges of the posterior advancement of the posterior cervical flap may create step deformities of the hairline, and certainly in those patients with extreme amounts of redundant skin, it does. In the typical case, the step of the hairline can be prevented or sufficiently minimized at closure by placing the suture bites greater or lesser distances apart, which pulls the superior edge of the wound sufficiently posterior to minimize the step and approximate the hairline of the posterior rotation of the posterior cervical flap. Even at their greatest, step deformities of the hairline rarely, if ever, are a source of complaint.

Postauricular Trimming of the Skin

The amount of skin trimmed in the postauricular area should be the smallest amount removed from any area, and at times is minimal or no trimming is

Figure 6–4. The placement of the initial occipital suture. **A.** Illustration of photograph (B). **B.** Intraoperative.

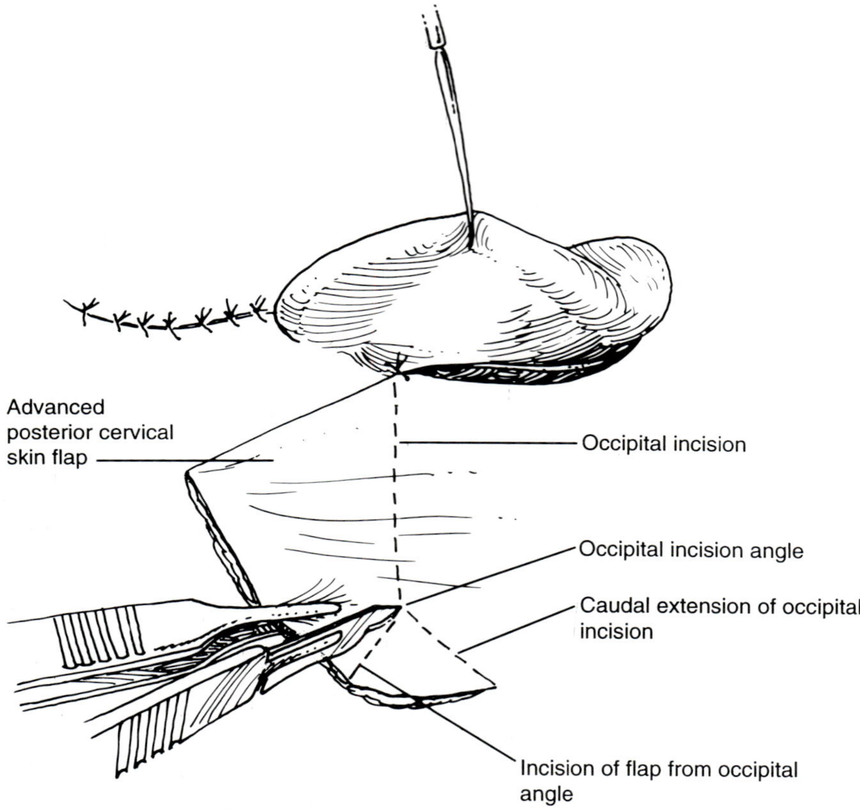

A

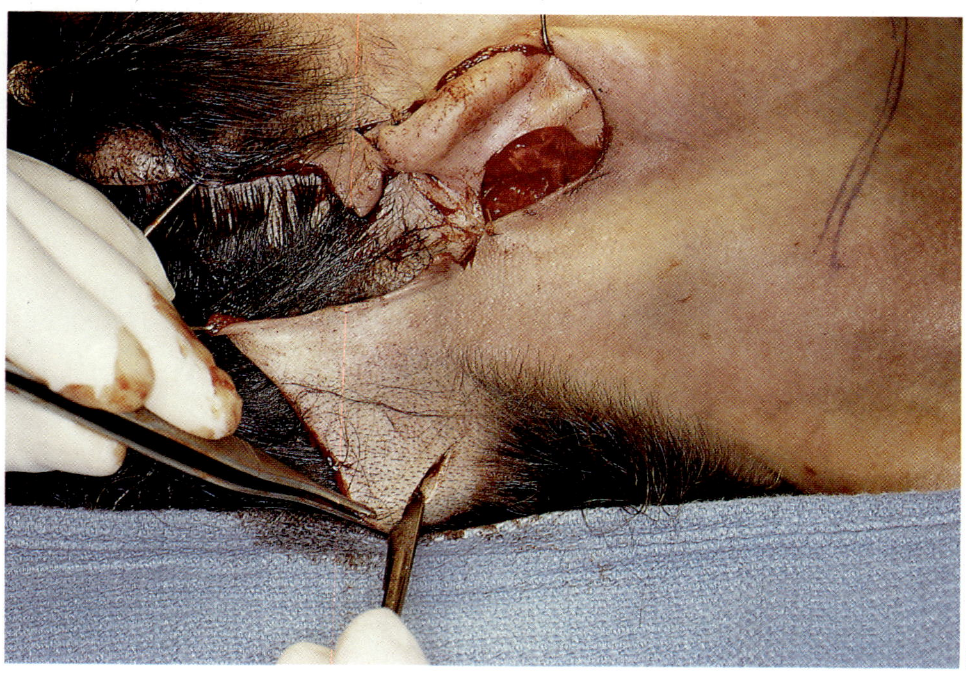

B

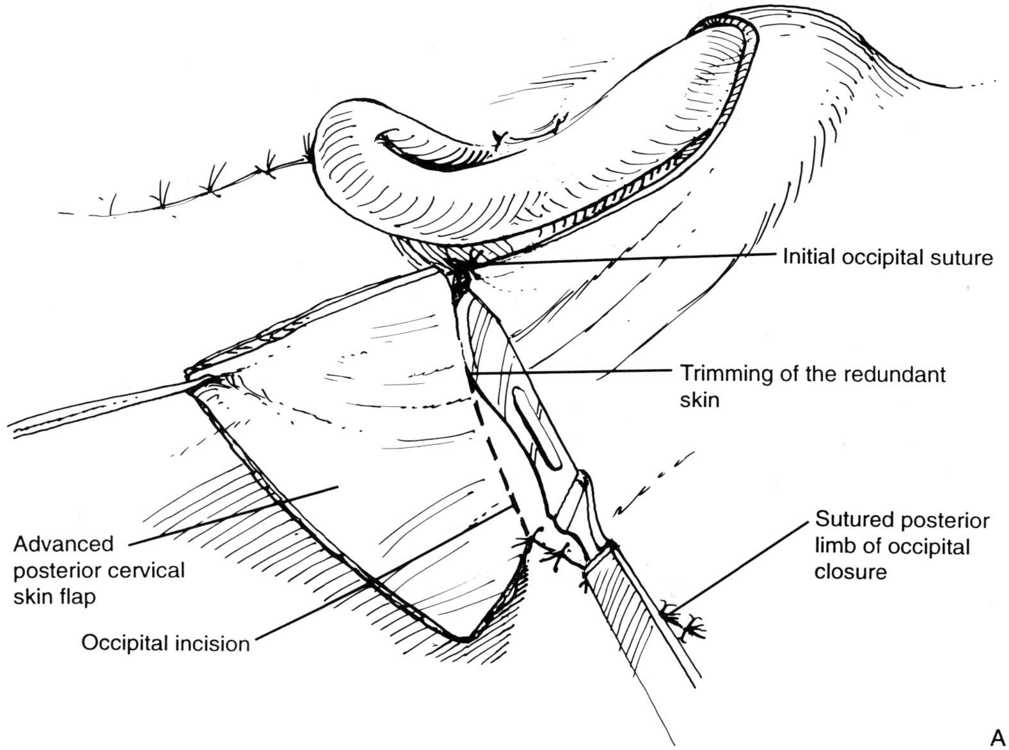

A

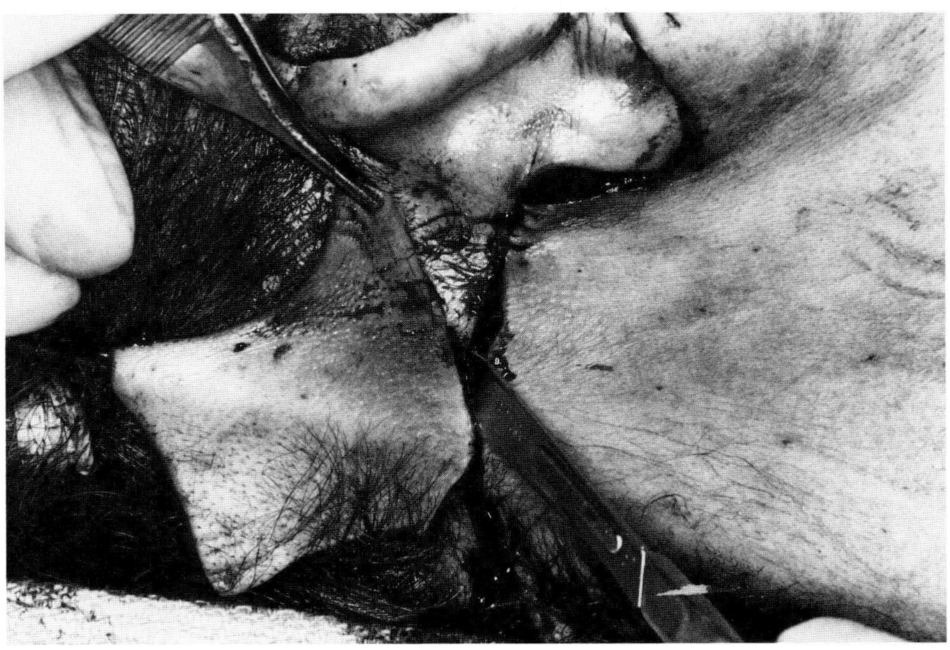

B

Figure 6–5. Trimming of the redundant posterior cervical skin flap. **A.** Illustration of photograph (B). **B.** Intraoperative.

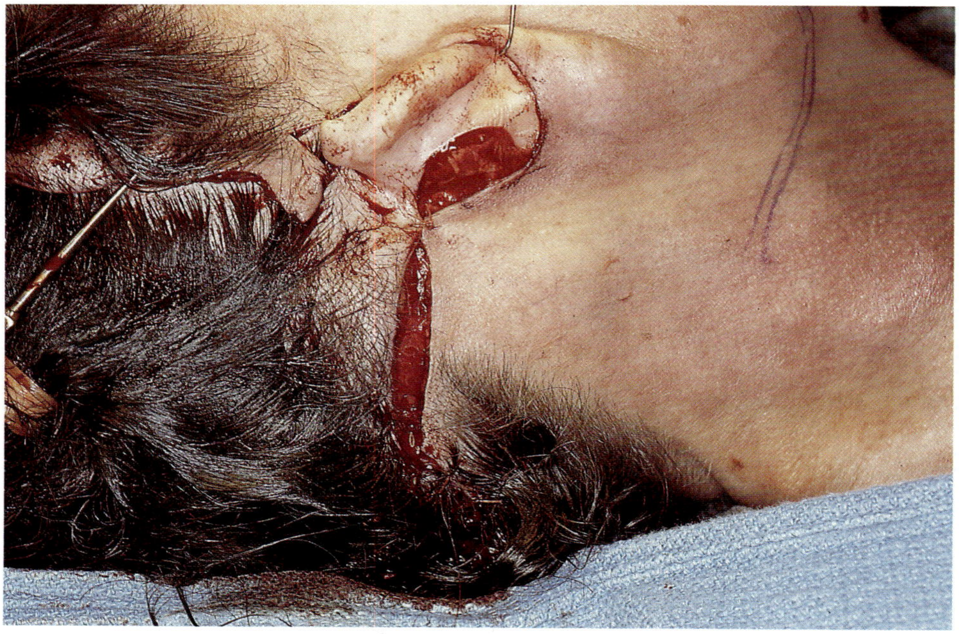

Figure 6–6. After trimming, the occipital wound edges are separated by approximately 1 cm.

required. If the direction of the posterior cervical flap is not directed more posteriorly during closure of the occipital limb of the wound, the flap is advanced anteriorly, which results in a large amount of skin in the postauricular sulcus. If this occurs, along with compression ("bunching") of the skin below the earlobe, the flap should be taken down and the direction adjusted more posteriorly. Otherwise, the compressed area will form permanent wrinkles just below the ear, which are very difficult to correct.

The ear is rolled anteriorly, being certain the earlobe is included. The trim of the skin flap behind the ear follows the posterior sulcus of the ear (Fig. 6–7), and is about 4 to 5 mm posterior to the sulcus. In Fig. 6–8, the posterior sulcus is highlighted by reflected light and the skin edge is a few millimeters posterior to the sulcus. The excess skin is trimmed best with serrated blade scissors.*

The trimming proceeds to the earlobe where it stops slightly short (cephalad) of the level of the lobule of the ear sulcus on the neck skin (see Fig. 6–8). At this point, the direction of the trim is curved anteriorly, creating the posterior half of the curvature for insertion of the earlobe. If the postauricular trim proceeds to the sulcus of the earlobe, the level of the curvature for insertion of the earlobe will drop further caudad after the preauricular trimming. Increased scarring and/or caudad traction on the earlobe may result.

The postauricular wound is not closed until all the trimming of the skin about the ear is complete. When it is closed, only a few interrupted 3–0 catgut (no. 822, Ethicon) sutures are necessary. If there is more than the usual bleeding, the wound can be left open until the left side of the face is completed. At the time of the application of the dressing, any collection of blood can be evacuated. The wound is then closed and the dressing applied.

*Kaye Face Lift Scissors, 7″ curved, serrated blades, Snowden-Pencer, Inc., Tucker, GA 30084.

Figure 6–7. Trimming of the redundant postauricular skin. **A.** Illustration of photograph (B). **B.** Intraoperative.

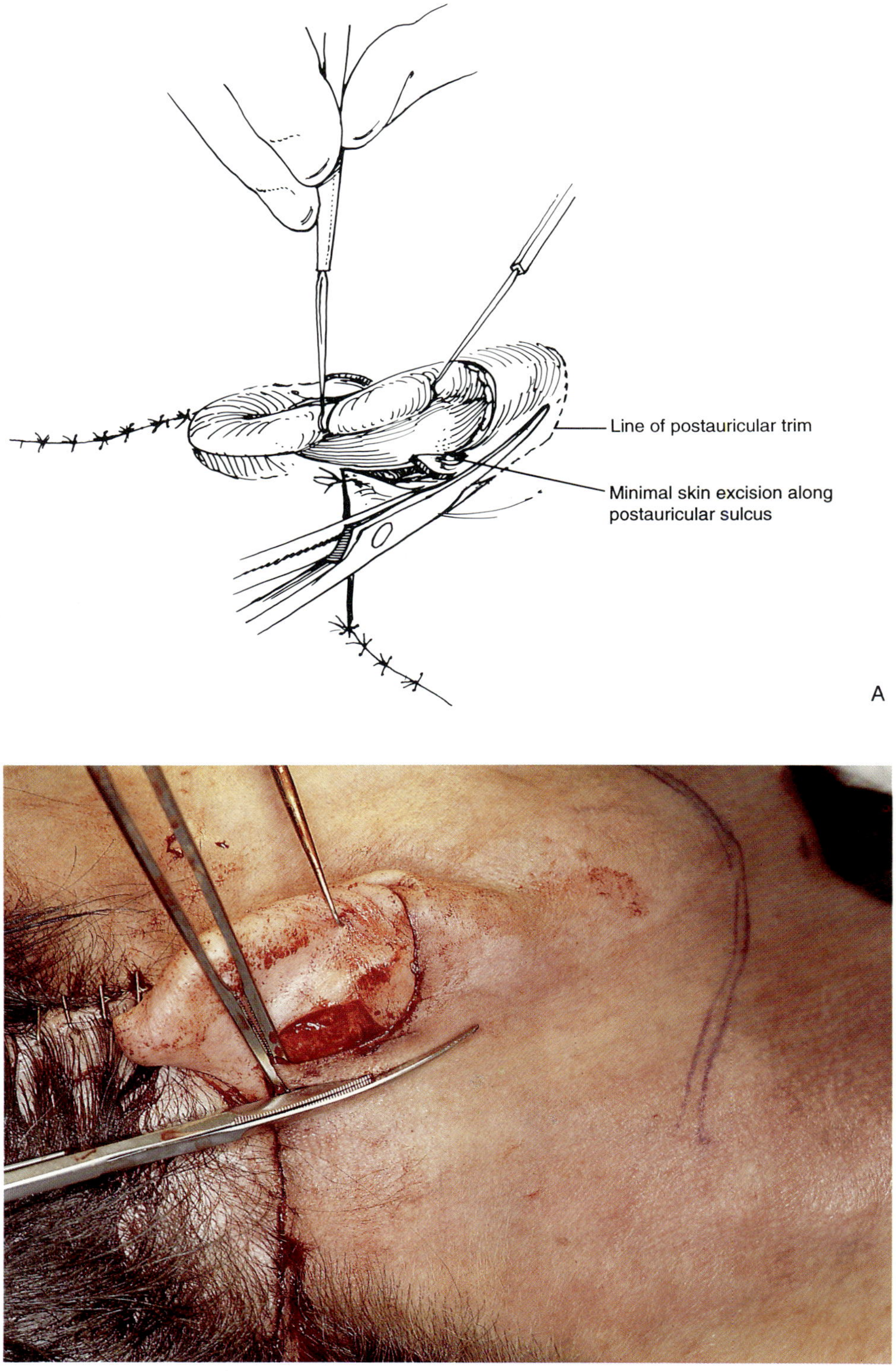

Figure 6–8. Cessation of postauricular skin trimming just above the lobule of the ear sulcus. **A.** Illustration of photograph (B). **B.** Intraoperative.

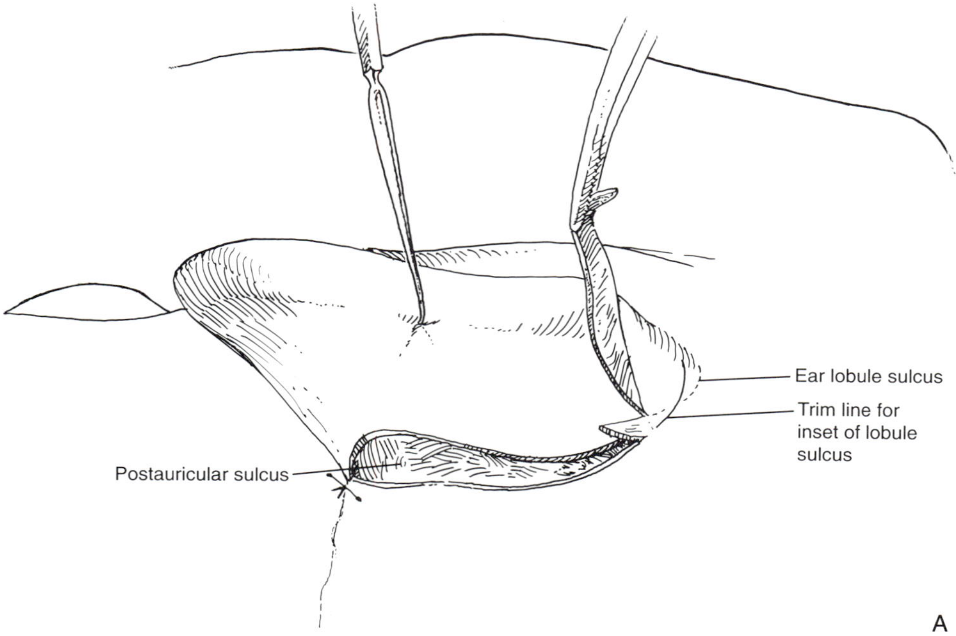

A

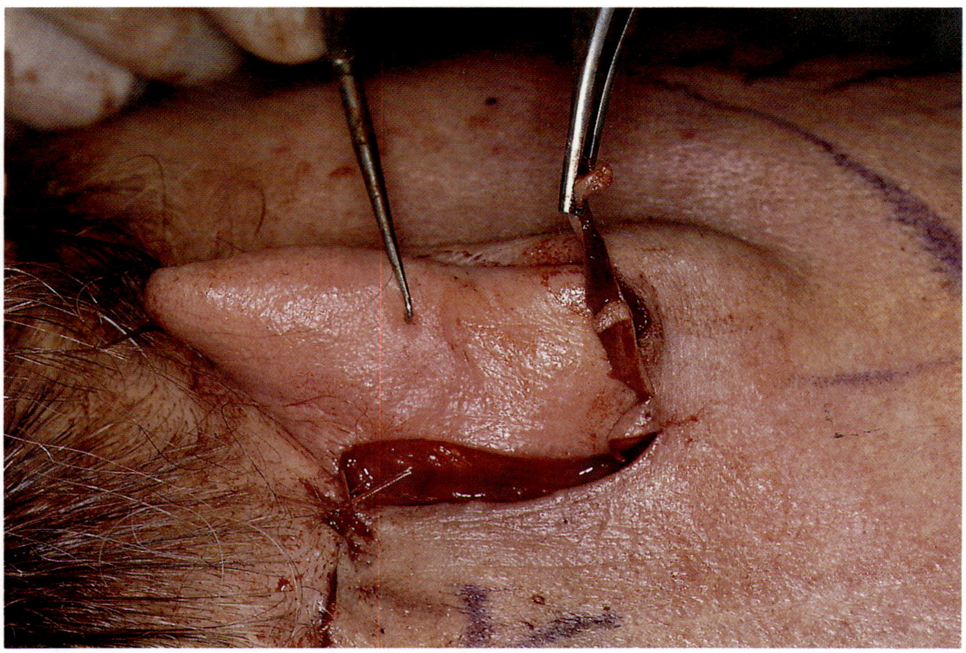

B

Preauricular Trimming of the Skin

The redrape of the skin of the cheek and preauricular region has no tension placed upon it. The support of the SMAS–platysma muscle (compound morphological unit) advancement and closure of the temporal and occipital limbs of the rhytidoplasty wound relieve any tension of the skin draping of the cheek; conversely, the preauricular wound closure is not a support area for the skin redraping. The cheek skin is massaged posteriorly with scissor blades or the hand to be certain the redraping is spread smoothly over the underlying tissues, and the scissors utilized to carefully trim the redundant skin. (Scissors with serrated blades provide the smoothest and most accurate trim.) The trim line follows the contours of the preauricular incision (Fig. 6–9) and is approximately 2 to 3 mm anterior to it (Fig. 6–10).

With the patient in the supine position, the earlobe falls posteriorly and when trimming the preauricular skin along the lobe segment, compensation should be made for this (see Fig. 6–10).

The removal of the excess skin of the cheek and the postauricular area inserts the ear in its normal position and without tension (see Fig. 6–10). The wound edges lie only a few millimeters apart and are easily approximated (5–0 nylon, no. 1666, Ethicon), which upon healing results in a very satisfactory fine line scar.

Skin Trimming in Tragus Rim Technique

When the tragus rim incision is employed, the skin trimming is executed in segments. The helix segment is removed to the superior border of the tragus, and the earlobe segment is removed from the inferior border of the tragus to the earlobe and joins the postauricular trim line. This leaves a "tongue" of skin (Fig. 6–11) covering the tragus. The pretragal skin is pressed into the cheek firmly to obliterate any tenting over the surface of the tragus and the tongue of tissue is trimmed along the tragus rim incision. The skin trimming of the pretragal flap ("tongue") should leave some excess length as with defatting of the dermis of the flap; the length of the concavity of the anterior surface of the tragus and the pretragal removal of fat may be longer than the trimmed flap. If the length of the insert of pretragal skin is too short, the tragus may be pulled forward and may expose the auditory canal.

Dermal Defatting of the Tragal Skin Flap

After the pretragal skin has been trimmed, the excess tissue and fat of the dermis of the tragus skin flap insert is excised from the undersurface of the skin until the dermis is cleared of any bulk that may obscure the sculptured contour of the tragus (Fig. 6–12). In effect, it is similar to a free full-thickness skin graft trimming of the dermis, but is a quadrilateral flap based medially. On occasion, if the defatting of the flap is too vigorous, there may be some necrosis. The objective is to provide as sculptured a tragus as possible, in spite of the fact that the advanced skin of the cheek is thicker than the original

Figure 6–9. Trimming of the redundant preauricular skin. **A.** Illustration of photograph (B). **B.** Intraoperative.

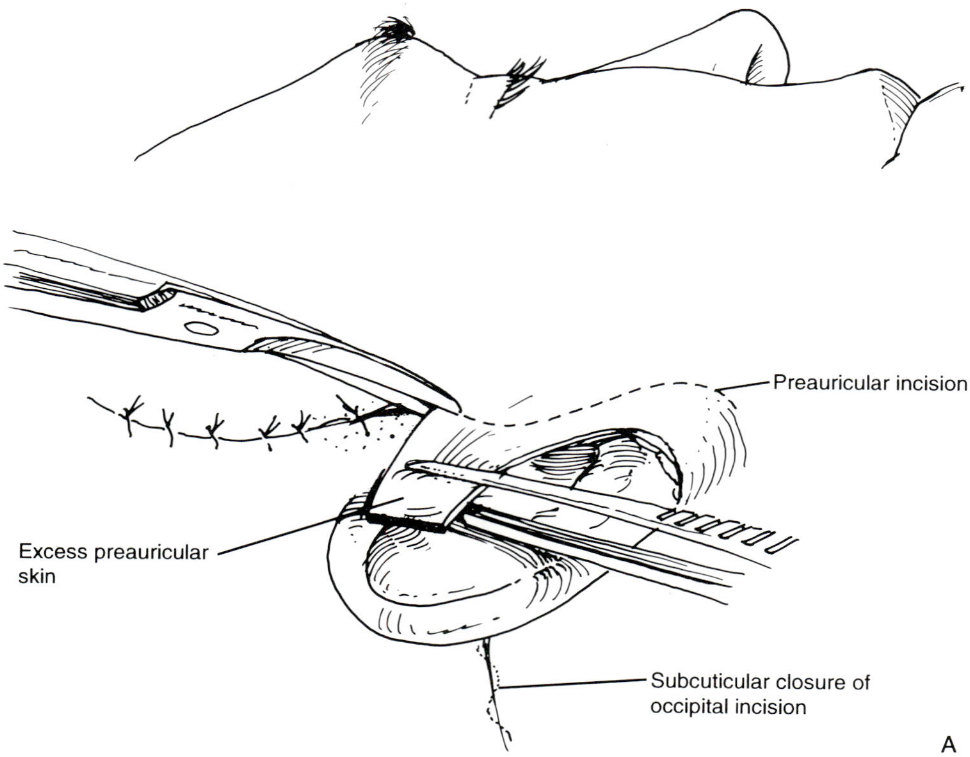

A

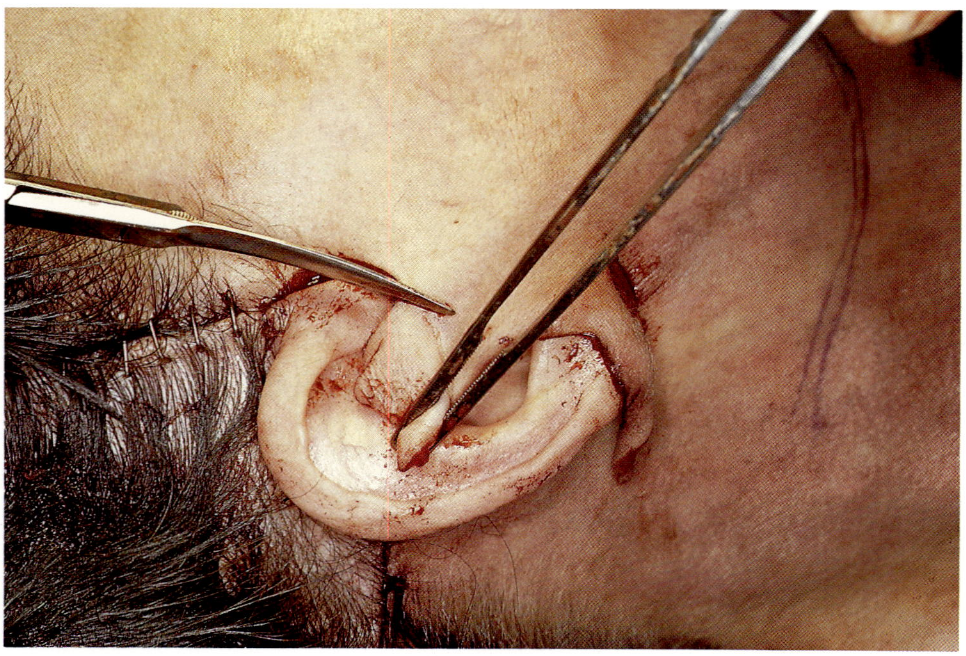

B

Figure 6–10. Skin edges separated 2 to 3 mm after preauricular skin trimming. **A.** Intraoperative.

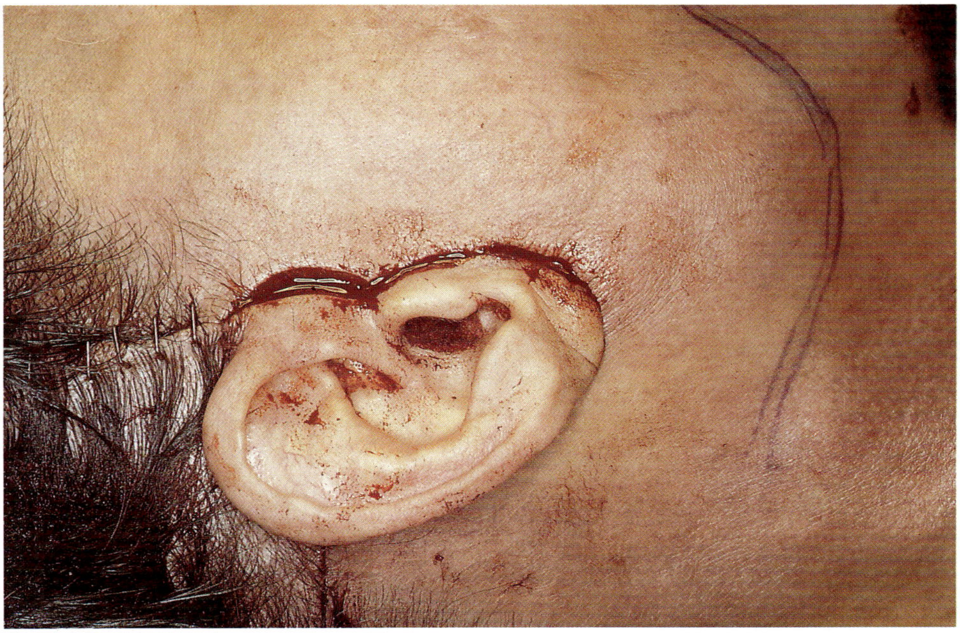

A

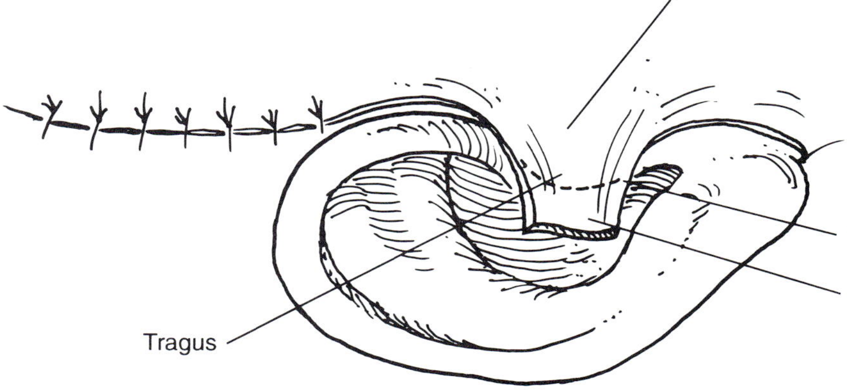

Figure 6–11. Trimming of the redundant preauricular skin with a tragus rim incision.

Figure 6–12. Defatting of the tragal skin insert. **A.** Illustration of photograph (B). **B.** Intraoperative.

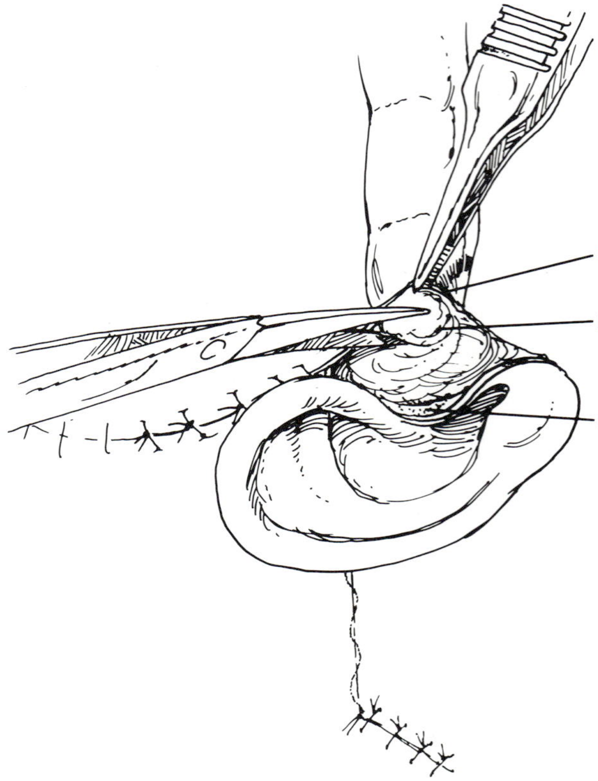

A

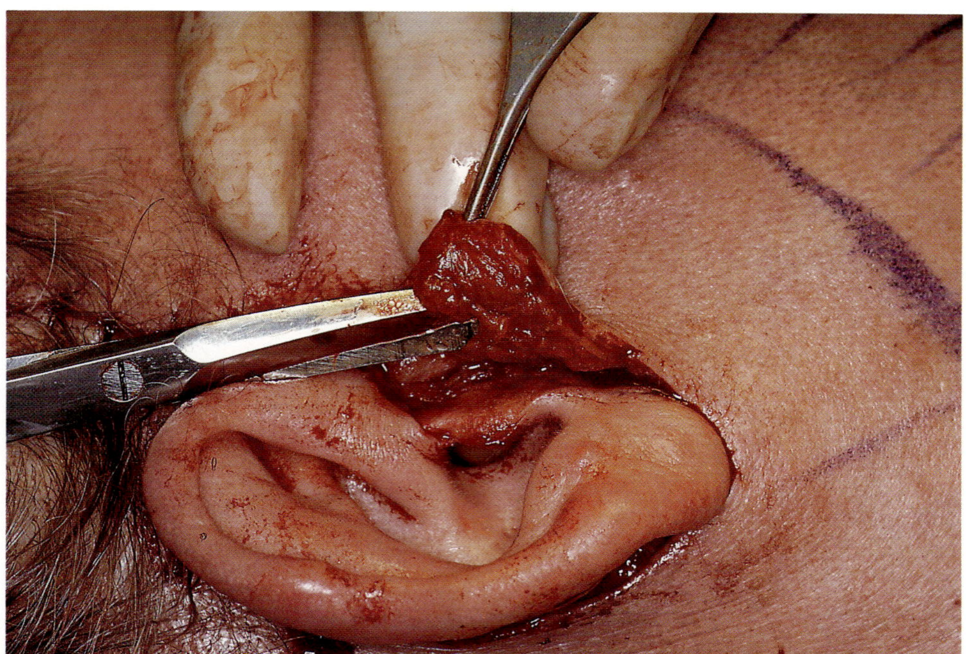

B

skin of the tragus. Again, the skin flap to be inserted on the tragus should be of sufficient length to mold to the tragus and still be slightly longer than necessary to allow for any contracture.

Sutured Preauricular and Postauricular Wound

The preauricular and postauricular wounds are closed (Fig. 6–13). The preauricular wound is approximated with interrupted 5–0 nylon suture (no. 1666, Ethicon). The postauricular wound is closed with interrupted 3–0 plain catgut. Plain catgut sutures cause very little scarring in the postauricular area. Also, catgut sutures (and staples) in the hair permit the patient to return at his or her convenience after the nylon sutures of the preauricular wound are removed in 4 to 5 days. With daily hair shampoos, the catgut sutures will dissolve, which can be an advantage.

The initial skin suture in the preauricular wound is placed at the earlobe. This ensures that the earlobe is inserted at the proper level and without any distortion. Another suture can be placed just below the tragus, and the remainder of the wound is closed caudad to cephalad.

Postoperative Rhytidectomy Dressing

After the left-side closure is completed and prior to application of the dressing, all areas, mostly the right side of the face and neck, are examined for collections of blood or hematoma. The neck is massaged free of any collections and if the postauricular wound on the right has not been closed, it is closed. Drains are not used. Though it is a matter of personal preference, their use does not seem to alter the recovery to any extent, and does not provide adequate evacuation of blood in the case of hematoma formation.

The dressing materials consist of dressing gauze squares,* approximately 18 in. of elasticized net,** and 4-in. Kling bandages.*** The gauze dressing squares are fluffed out on the sterile field (Fig. 6–14A). Six to eight are unfolded one time and stacked. These are used across the forehead. All wounds are covered with Polysporin ointment, which makes the dressing less adherent and easier to remove. The antibiotic is probably not necessary as facial wounds seldom become infected; however, if a wound did become infected, it might be difficult to explain why some antibiotic ointment was not used.

The first step in application of the dressing is to stretch out a single, opened, fluffed gauze square and place it in the postauricular sulcus, bringing it around the earlobe and packing it into the concha. When the postauricular surface and the concha are packed sufficiently (two to three pieces) to maintain the ear in its usual position, a handful of gauze fluffs are placed

---

*Kendall Curity, 4″ × 4″. The Kendall Co., Kendall Health Care Products, Mansfield, MA 02048.
**Flexinet, Genetic Laboratories, Inc., St. Paul, MN 55113.
***Kling, 4″. Johnson & Johnson Medical, Inc., Arlington, TX 76004-0130.

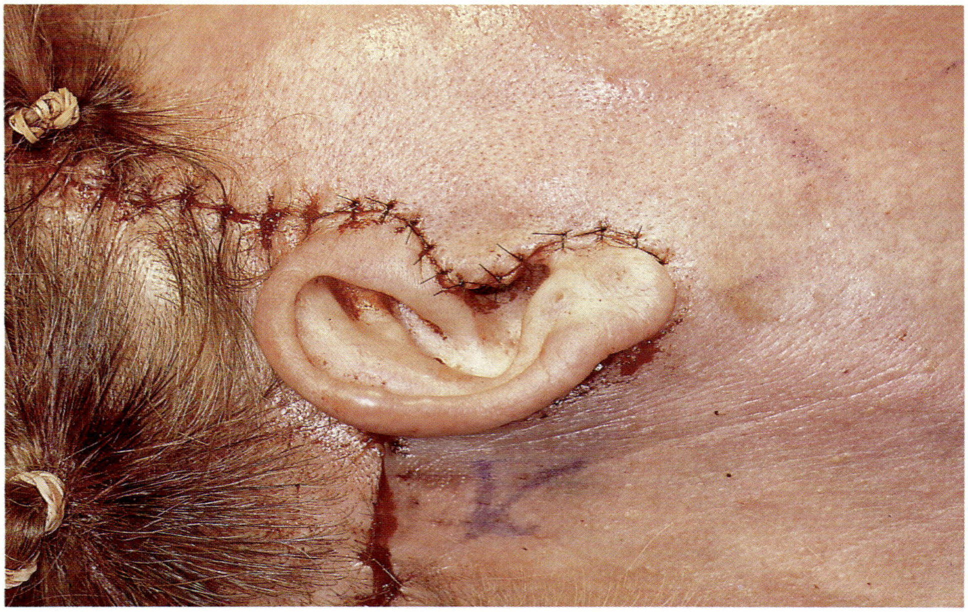

A

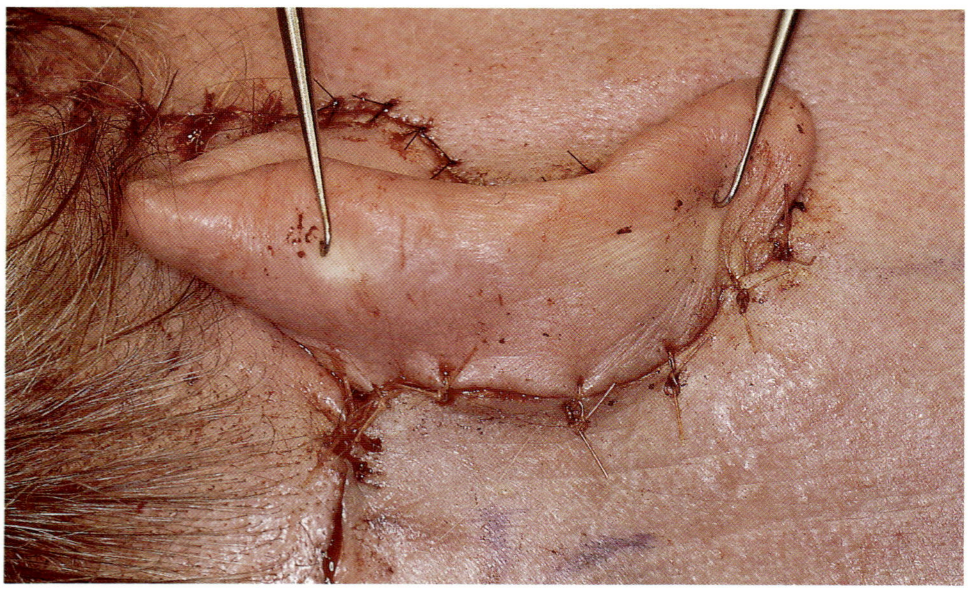

B

Figure 6–13. Completed preauricular and postauricular wound closure. **A.** Preauricular, intraoperative. **B.** Postauricular, intraoperative.

over the ear as if it were an earmuff. The dressing of the ears is held in place and another handful of fluffs are placed over the occipital areas. A large number of fluffs are now placed in the submental area and the anterior cervical region. It is particularly important that there be a large amount of bulk on the anterior portion of the neck and the submental area. This, and no pillow under the head postoperatively, will help prevent flexion of the neck anteriorly. If the head is flexed, it may cause advancement of the skin into the submental region, which may create a permanent skin fold in the submental area posterior to the submental incision and mar an otherwise superior result.

Figure 6–14. Rhytidectomy head dressing. **A.** Fluffed dressing gauze squares. **B.** Dressing applied.

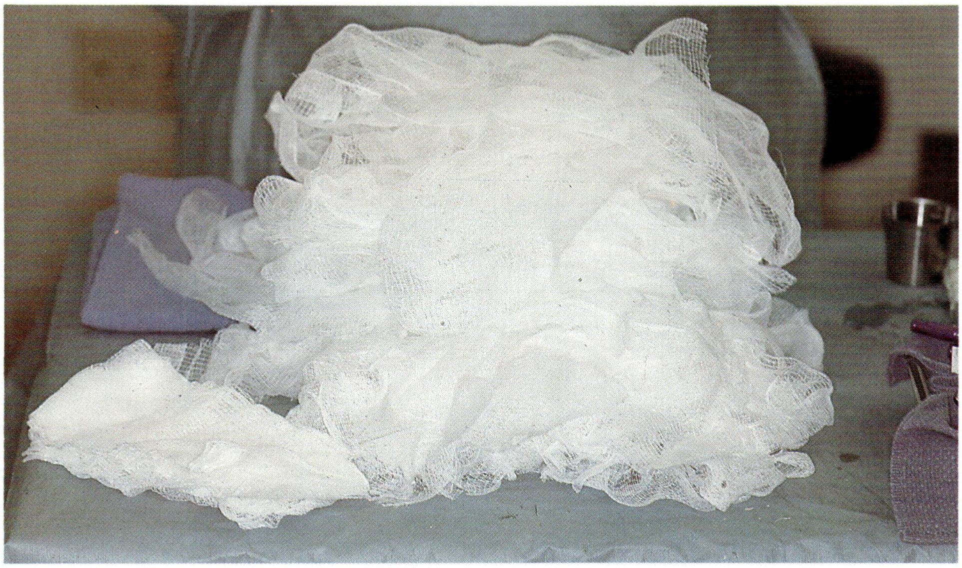

A

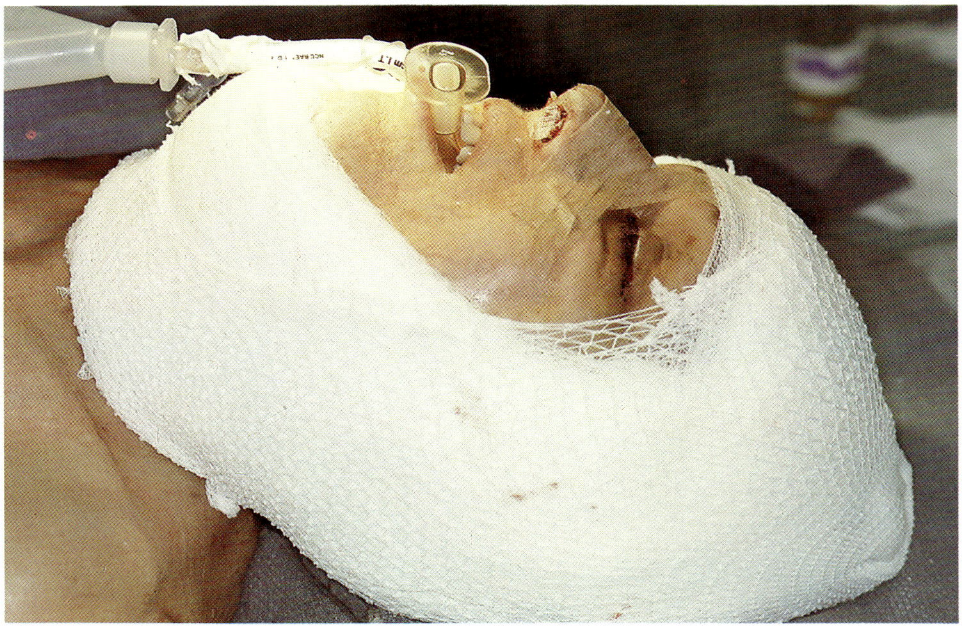

B

The gauze dressing squares, opened one fold, are placed on the forehead. Four-inch Kling gauze dressings are applied from the vertex to the submental region and about the head until moderate compression is achieved over the entire area. A piece of flexible net tubular dressing, approximately 18 in. long, is brought over the head, the anesthesia tubes are disconnected, and the dressing is pulled well down on the neck. The remaining length of tubular net dressing at the vertex is twisted and brought over the head in a similar manner. The face area is opened and the patient is prepared for transfer to a recovery area when the anesthesia department is satisfied with the patient's condition (see Fig. 6–14B).

The head dressing is removed the day after surgery.

SEVEN

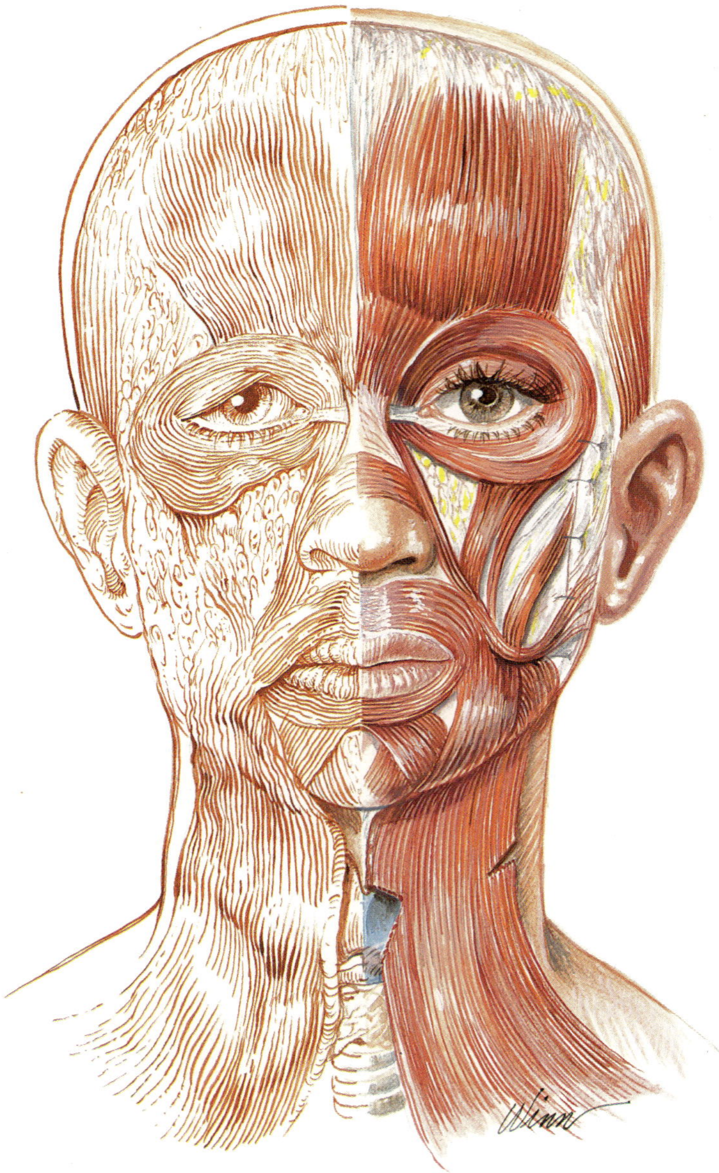

SMAS-Platysma Muscle Rhytidectomy Cases

Rather than present ideal case results, which can be done for almost every rhytidectomy technique, five cases have been chosen to demonstrate the results possible in patients with advanced changes of the skin and the underlying SMAS and musculature of the face and neck, and to show that the techniques described in the preceding chapters can permanently maintain improvement, or at least stabilize and slow the progress of recurring aging disharmony of the face and neck for long periods of time even though the changes are more advanced. Postoperative results are influenced by severe aging changes, but the cases with more advanced changes give credence to the SMAS-platysma muscle, and platysma muscle of the submental region restoration with varying degrees of lipectomy procedure.

Cases 1 and 2 present severe atrophic skin changes with marked cutis laxa and platysma muscle folds in which there is no excess subcutaneous fat and the underlying cervicomental angle is satisfactory. Case 3 presents marked cutis laxa with prominent nasolabial folds and thin platysma folds of the neck. The underlying cervicomental angle is satisfactory. The durations of patient follow-up in Cases 1 through 3 are 4 months, 7 years, and 12 years, respectively.

Cases 4 and 5 illustrate patients who present with marked cutis laxa of the face and neck, an obtuse cervicomental angle, and a midline skin and fat fold of the neck and who may or may not have hypogenesis of the mentum. The durations of patient follow-up in Cases 4 and 5 are 6 months and 6 years, respectively.

Cutis Laxa of the Face and Neck, Satisfactory Cervicomental Angle, and Platysma Muscle Folds of the Neck

Case 1

Findings

A 58-year-old female (Fig. 7–1A,C,E) had marked cutis laxa of the face and neck. There were deep wrinkles of the cheeks lateral to the oral commissures and increased prominence of the nasolabial folds. The jaw showed minimal jowl formation. The platysma muscle folds were prominent, but the underlying cervicomental angle and mandible line were good.

Intraoperative Sequence of the Rhytidectomy

1. Submental area (see Chapter 3):
   a. Subdermal skin elevation.
   b. Resection/approximation of the redundant anterior borders of the platysma muscle.
   c. Wedge resection of the anterior border of the platysma muscle at the cervicomental level.
   d. No fat removal.
2. Temporal region: Elevation of the superficial temporal fascia (see Chapter 4).
3. Cheek and posterior cervical region: Subdermal elevation of skin flaps (see Chapter 4).
4. Cheek SMAS and medial subcutaneous dissection of infraorital area (zygomatic zone) (see Chapter 5): Extensive elevation to the nasolabial fold.
5. Skin redrape and closure (see Chapter 6).

Discussion

Postoperatively (Fig. 7–1B,D,F), the SMAS restoration reduced the depth of the nasolabial folds and improved the appearance of the marked atrophic skin changes and wrinkling of the cheeks. The release of the SMAS in the tightly adherent area of the malar prominence provided a good redrape of the area. The "swag" of the lower eyelid and descent of the skin in the malar region have been corrected. This combined with the lower blepharoplasty produces the young appearance desired. (There was no upper blepharoplasty. The lower lid blepharoplasty and brow lift add further to the overall harmony.)

The thin platysma muscle folds were corrected by resection of the anterior borders of the platysma and approximation by advancing (tightening) the platysma in the submental and submandibular region. A moderate (2.5–3.0-cm) wedge/transection of the anterior border of the platysma muscle at the level of the cervicomental angle provides stability at the angle. The redrape of the skin of the neck relieved the skin relaxation of the neck, minimizing the

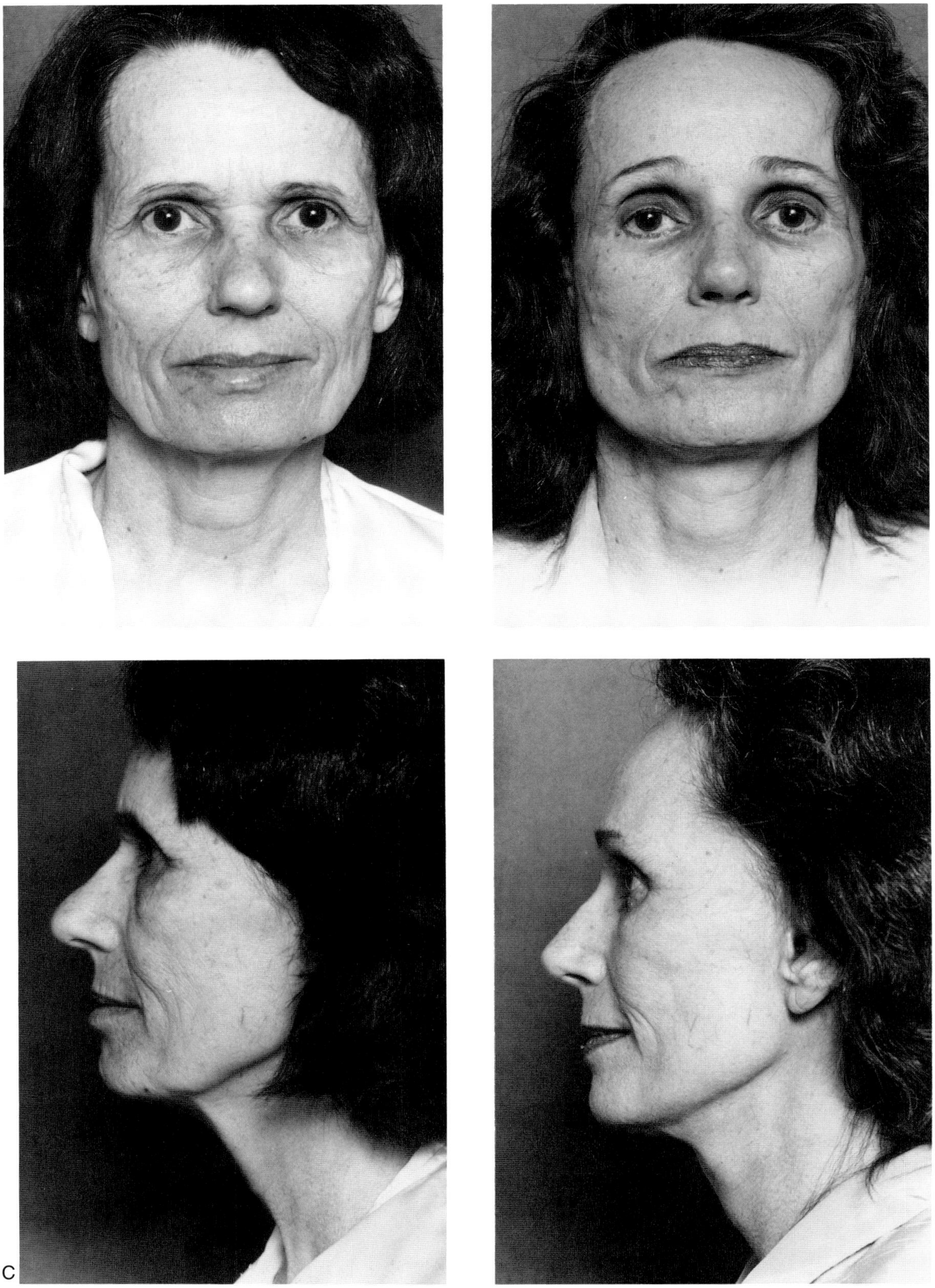

A B C D

Figure 7–1. A 58-year-old female. **A,C,E.** Before rhytidectomy (1990). **B,D,F.** After rhytidectomy (4 months).

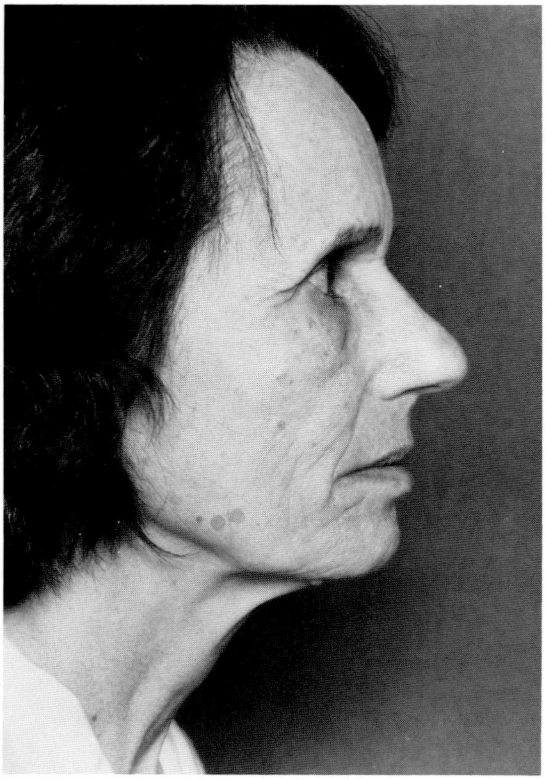

E

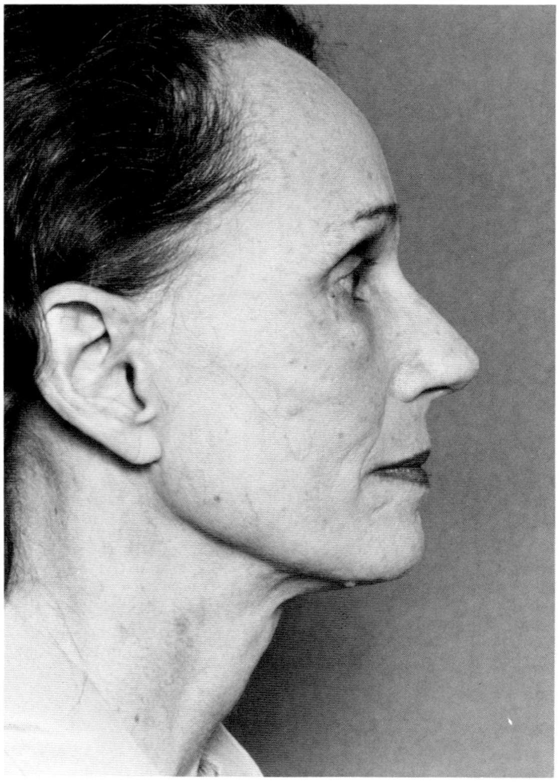

F

Figure 7–1 (continued)

midneck crease. The anterior borders of the platysma below the cervicomental angle are lateral to the structures of the anterior region of the neck in a more normal relationship, as seen in the preoperative view of the lower portion of the neck. The cervicomental wedge/transection relieved the tension on the muscle. The neck appears normal and young.

The nasal tip changes are outlined in Chapter 8.

Case 2

Findings

A 61-year-old female (Fig. 7–2) had severe cutis laxa of the face and neck. There were marked actinic skin changes with prominent permanent wrinkles of the cheeks and perioral region, greater on the left side than on the right. Deepening of the nasolabial folds was greater on the left than on the right. She had minimal to moderate jowl formation and severe actinic skin changes of the neck. There were marked thin skin–platysma muscle folds, and the underlying cervicomental angle and mandible line were satisfactory.

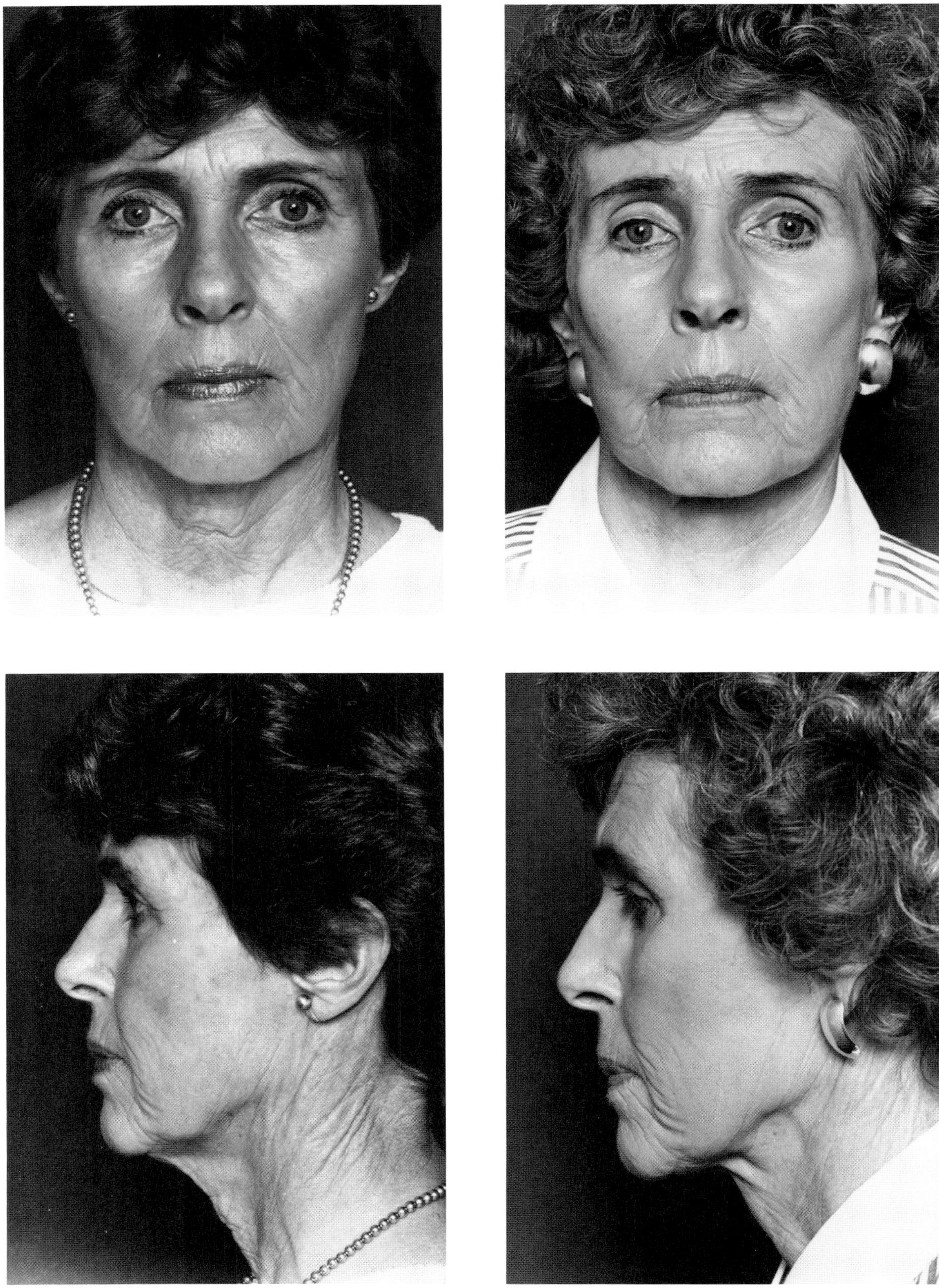

A B C D

Figure 7–2. A 61-year-old female. **A,C,E.** Before rhytidectomy (1985). **B,D,F.** After rhytidectomy (7 years).

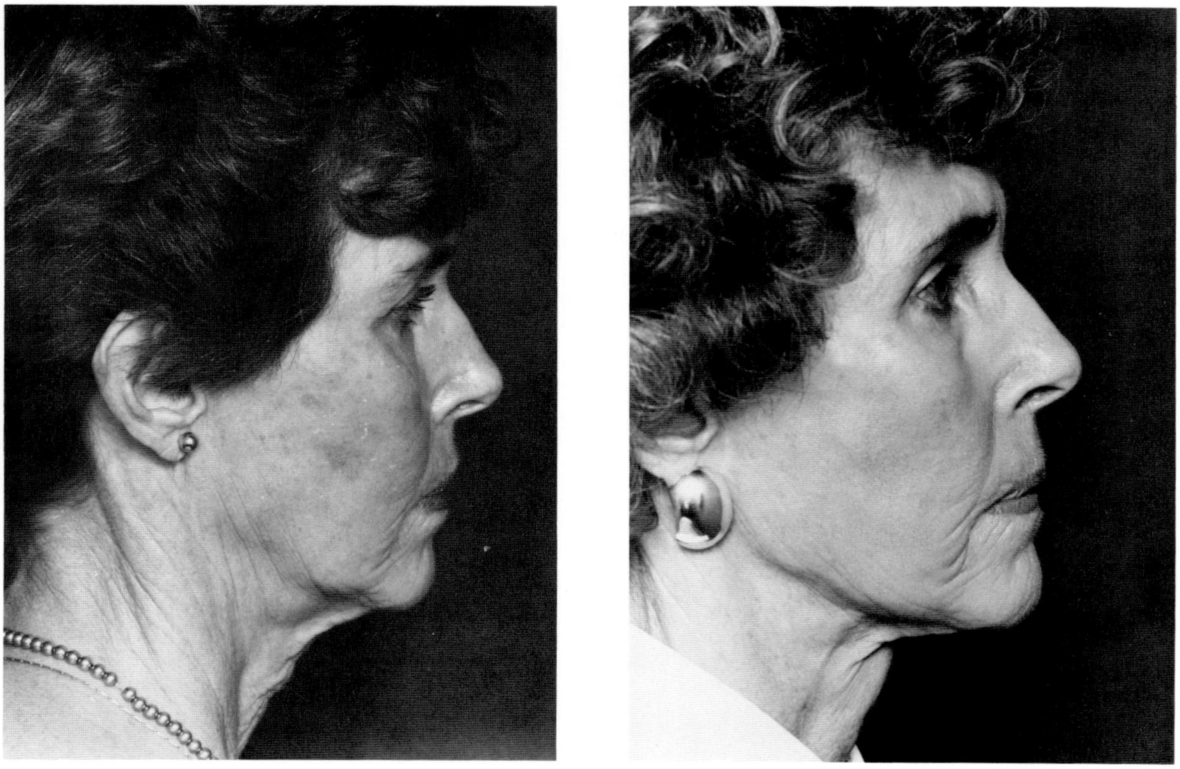

E F

Figure 7–2 (continued)

INTRAOPERATIVE SEQUENCE OF THE RHYTIDECTOMY

1. Submental area (see Chapter 3):
   a. Elevation of skin and subcutaneous fat.
   b. Minimal lipectomy of the jowl and the submental area.
   c. Resection/approximation of the anterior border of the platysma muscle.
   d. Wedge resection of the anterior border of the platysma muscle at the cervicomental angle level.
2. Temporal area: Elevation of the superficial temporal fascia (see Chapter 4).
3. Cheek and posterior cervical region: Subdermal elevation of skin flaps (see Chapter 4).
4. Cheek SMAS and medial subcutaneous dissection of the infraorbital area (zygomatic zone) (see Chapter 5): Extensive elevation with penetration to the nasolabial fold.
5. Skin redrape and closure (see Chapter 6).

Discussion

The extensive release of the SMAS reduced the nasolabial folds, which at 7 years postoperatively (Fig. 7–2B,D,F) appeared better than the preoperative appearance in the frontal view. The lateral view shows that the nasolabial fold is stable, appearing less defined than preoperatively in spite of the marked increase in the wrinkling of the lower portion of the fold and the area below the oral commissure. The jawline on the right maintained good contour, whereas on the left an early jowl was noticeable.

In the neck, the platysma muscle restoration in the submental region and the cervicomental wedge/transection (moderate), along with the skin redrape, maintained a satisfactory appearance of the area and eliminated the fine wrinkling of the skin of the neck.

Case 3

Findings

A 48-year-old female (Fig. 7–3A,C,E) had moderate cutis laxa of the face and neck. The skin of the cheeks was relaxed and the nasolabial folds were prominent. There was submalar depression, greater on the left than on the right. The mandible line was satisfactory except for jowl fat, particularly on

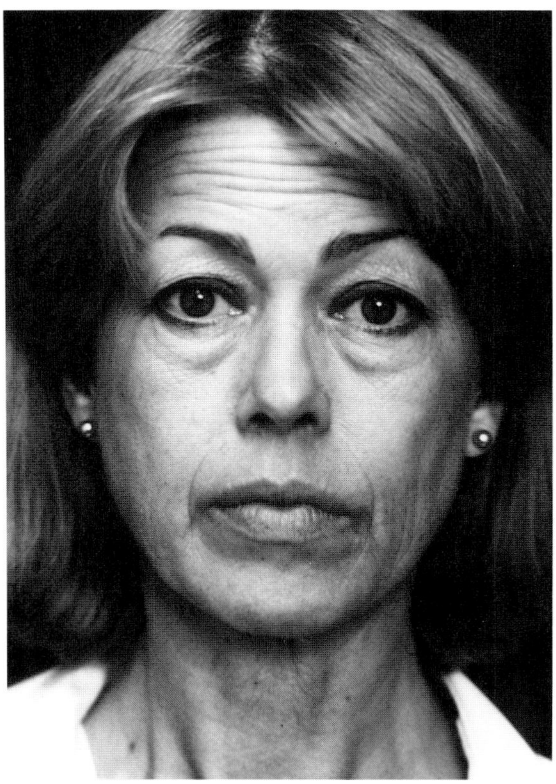
A

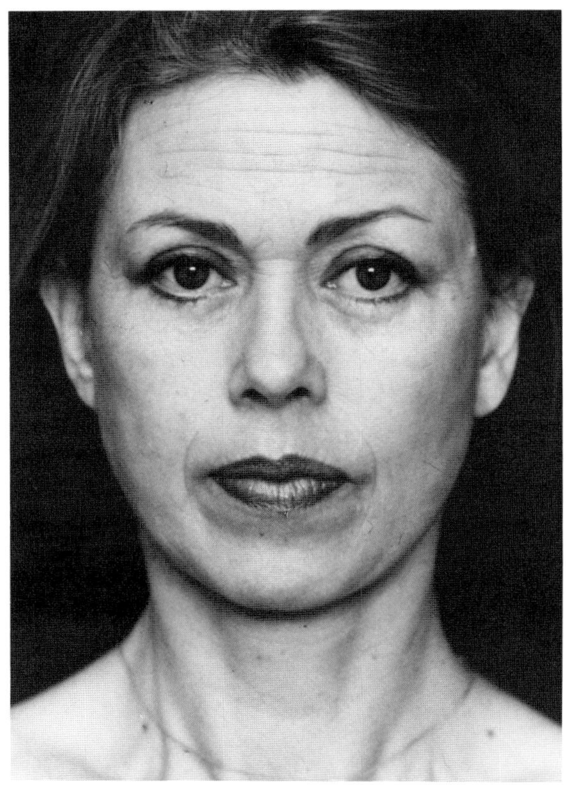
B

Figure 7–3. A 48-year-old female. **A,C,E.** Before rhytidectomy (1978). **B,D,F.** After rhytidectomy (2 years). **G,H,I.** After rhytidectomy (12 years).

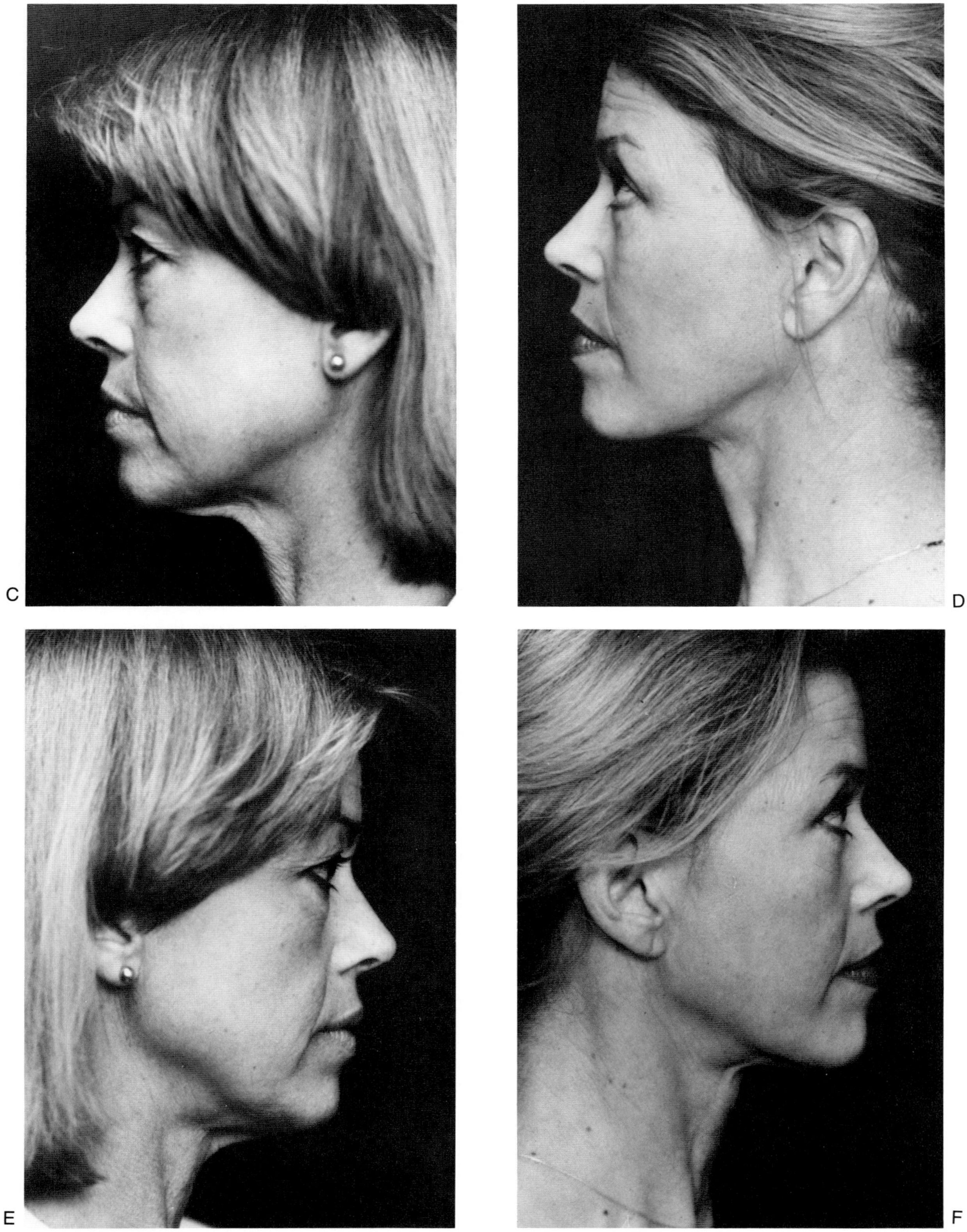

Figure 7–3 (continued)

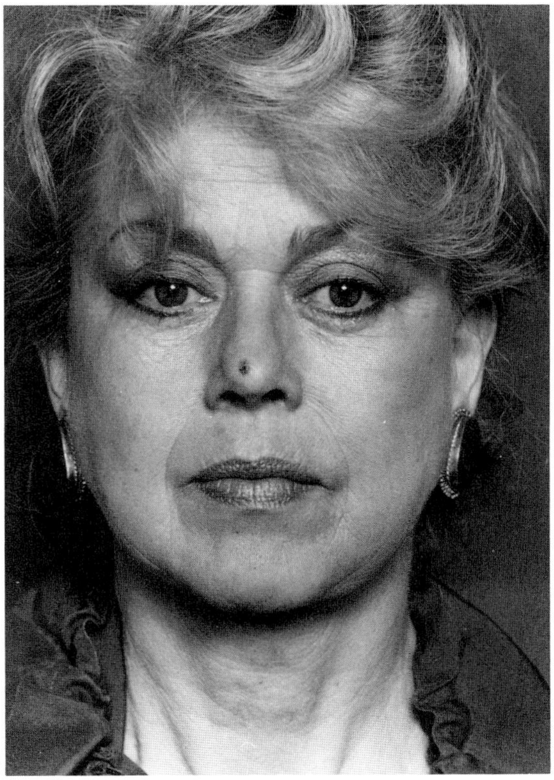

G

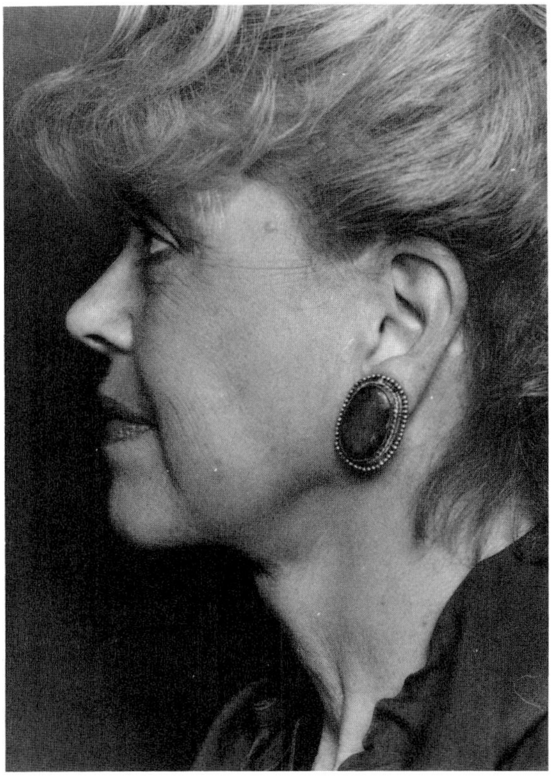

H

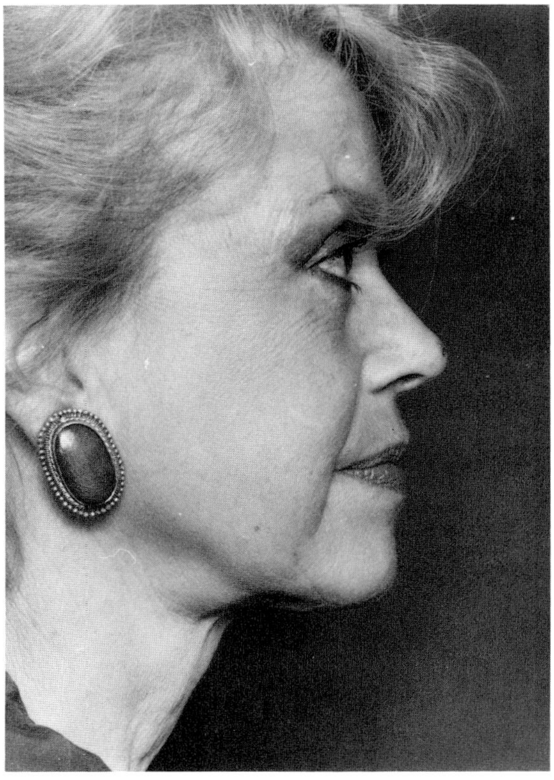

I

Figure 7–3 (continued)

the right side. The submandibular gland was distinguishable, greater on the right than on the left. (This should be pointed out to the patients as it influences short- and long-term results in this area.) There were thin platysma muscle folds of the submental region. The skin of the neck showed marked fine wrinkling. The subcutaneous fat layer was thin.

Intraoperative Sequence of the Rhytidectomy

1. Submental area (see Chapter 3).
   a. Skin and subcutaneous fat elevation.
   b. Resection/approximation of the anterior border of the platysma muscle.
   c. Wedge/subtotal transection of the platysma muscle, anterior two thirds, at the cervicomental angle.
2. Temporal region (see Chapter 4): Elevation of the superficial temporal fascia.
3. Cheek and posterior cervical region (see Chapter 4): Subdermal elevation of the skin flaps.
4. Cheek SMAS and medial subcutaneous dissection of the infraorbital area (zygomatic zone) (see Chapter 5): Extensive elevation with penetration to the nasolabial fold.
5. Skin redrape and closure (see Chapter 6).

Discussion

Two years postoperatively (Fig. 7–3B,D,F), the front view reveals good contours of the malar region. The submalar area depression (left) was obliterated. The release of the tightly adherent superficial and deep fasciae (or ligament) in the area provided the mobility for good restoration, and the younger appearance desired. At 12 years postoperatively (Fig. 7–3G,H,I) the result remained satisfactory.

The nasolabial folds and wrinkles of the cheek appeared greatly improved at 2 years postoperatively, and were more prominent at 12 years, but not a great deal more than preoperatively. (Some weight gain was observed at 12 years.) The jawline at 2 years maintained good contour. At 12 years, jowls, similar to the preoperative appearance, had recurred. The preoperatively prominent submandibular glands contributed, along with the skin relaxation, to the submandibular folds.

The neck restoration was maintained well at 2 and 12 years, which is a result of subtotal transection of the platysma muscle and resection of the anterior borders of the platysma muscle with approximation (anterior advancement) of the muscle in the submental region. The platysma folds and marked skin relaxation of the cervicomental angle were relieved (at 2 and 12 years postoperatively). The reduction of the wrinkling of the neck was maintained by a satisfactory redraping.

(The nasal tip lesion seen at the 12-year visit was a basal cell carcinoma.)

Cutis Laxa of the Face and Neck, Obtuse Cervicomental Angle, and Skin and Fat Folds of the Neck

Case 4

Findings

A 62-year-old female (Fig. 7–4A,C,E) had severe cutis laxa of the face and neck. The redundant skin of the cheeks deepened the nasolabial fold, which continued as a vertical skin fold across the mandible and through the submandibular area to the approximate level of the thyroid cartilage. The mandibular border was obscured by thick subcutaneous fat. Hypogenesis of the mentum was present. The neck had a large, fatty midline fold extending from the submental crease to just below the midneck crease (see Fig. 7–4A,C,E).

Intraoperative Sequence of the Rhytidectomy

1. Submental area (Chapter 3):
   a. Subcutaneous fat elevated at the preplatysma muscle level.
   b. Resection/approximation of the anterior borders of the platysma muscle.
   c. Approximately one-third of the subplatysma muscle fat excised as an inverted "V" wedge.
   d. Borders of fat wedge resection approximated.
   e. Anterior borders of the platysma muscle resected and approximated.
   f. Cervicomental wedge/transection of the platysma muscle (anterior) (approximately half width of the muscle).
   g. Submental fat pad excised.
   h. Limited liposuction of submandibular fat pad (jowl).
   i. Chin implant inserted (see Chapter 8).
2. Temporal region (see Chapter 4): Elevation of the superficial temporal fascia.
3. Cheek and posterior cervical region (see Chapter 4): Subdermal elevation of skin flaps.
4. Skin and subcutaneous fat elevation from sternomastoid muscle to join submental preplatysma muscle dissection (see Chapter 4).
5. Cheek SMAS elevation and medial subcutaneous dissection of the infraorbital area (zygomatic zone) (see Chapter 5): Extensive elevation to the nasolabial fold.
6. Skin redrape and closure (see Chapter 6).

Discussion

The postoperative rhytidectomy views (Fig. 7–4B,D,F) show the creation of a cervicomental angle (subplatysma muscle and submental lipectomy and a more extensive transection of the anterior border of the platysma). The subcutaneous fat layer was maintained at a thickness in harmony with the rest of

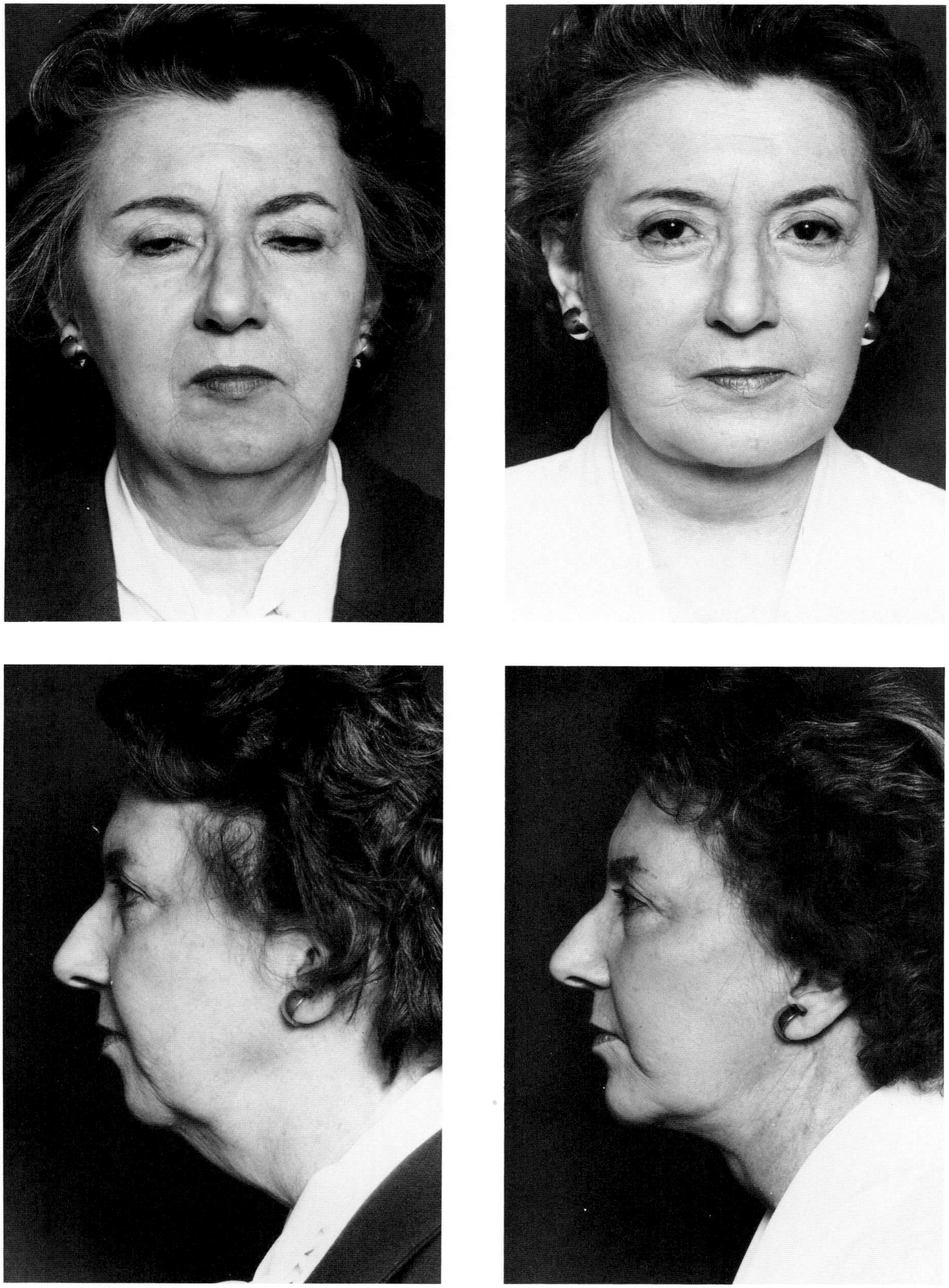

A B C D

Figure 7–4. A 62-year-old female. **A,C,E.** Before rhytidectomy (1991). **B,D,F.** After rhytidectomy (6 months).

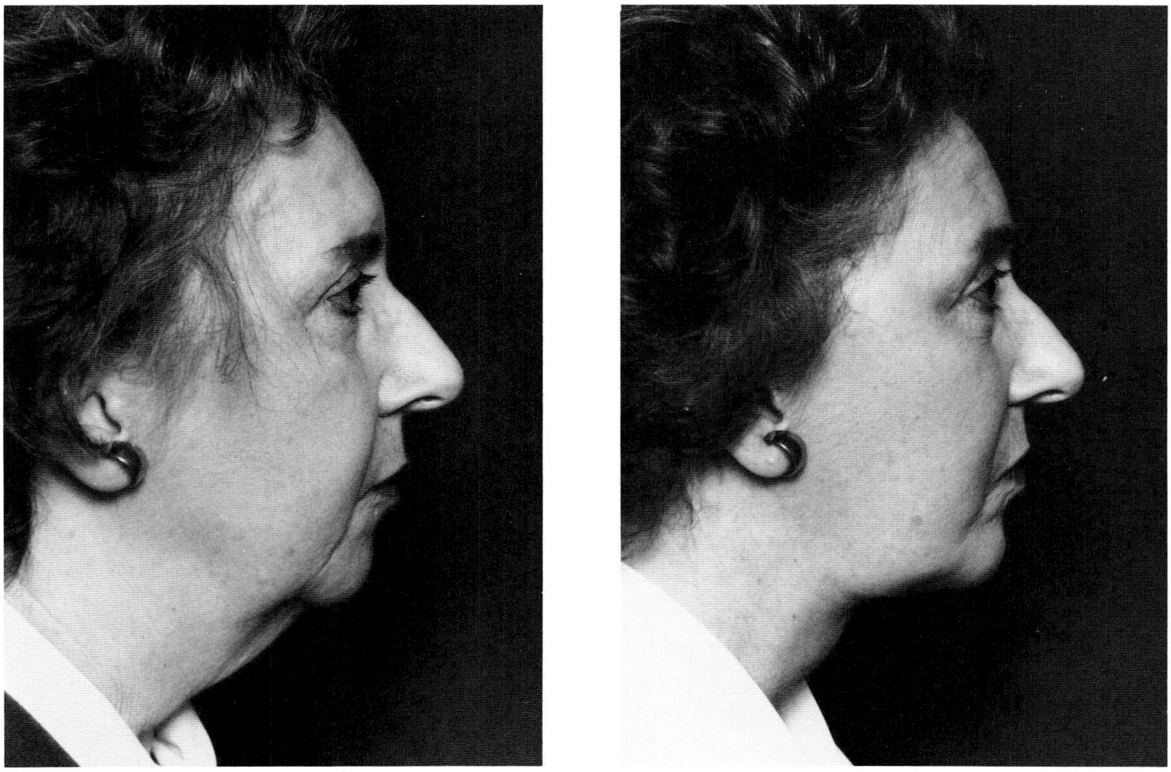

E F

Figure 7–4 (continued)

the face and neck. It is better to err on the side of leaving more fat as it will appear more normal postoperatively.

At a future time any excess fat can be pared down, and it is much simpler as the objective is more limited. The nasolabial folds that extended to the submandibular region were improved and a jawline established. This was aided by the chin implant. The overall result was quite satisfactory for the facies presenting with "heavy" fat cheeks, an obtuse cervicomental angle with a heavy fat skin fold of the neck, and hypogenesis of the mentum, all of which contributed to the loss of a mandibular line and cheek and jowl redundancy.

Case 5

Findings

A 55-year-old female (Fig. 7–5A,C,E) had severe cutis laxa of the face and neck. The redundant skin of the face deepened the nasolabial folds, which continued inferiorly, lateral to the oral commissure, across the mandible border, continuing on the neck to the level of the thyroid cartilage (left fold more prominent than right). The jawline was obscured. The neck had a large,

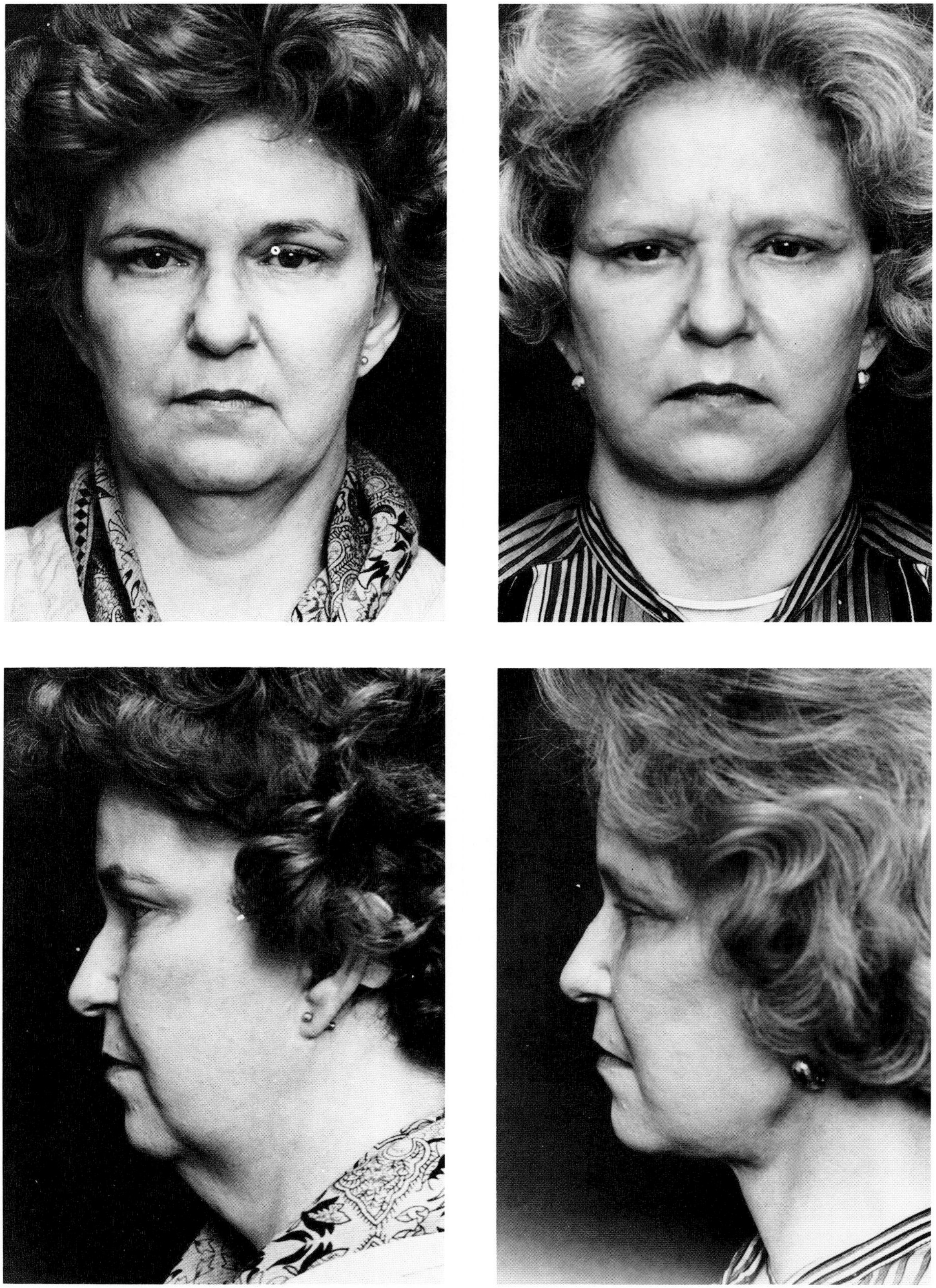

Figure 7–5. A 55-year-old female. **A,C,E.** Before rhytidectomy (1979). **B,D,F.** After rhytidectomy (6 months). **G,H,I.** After rhytidectomy (6 years).

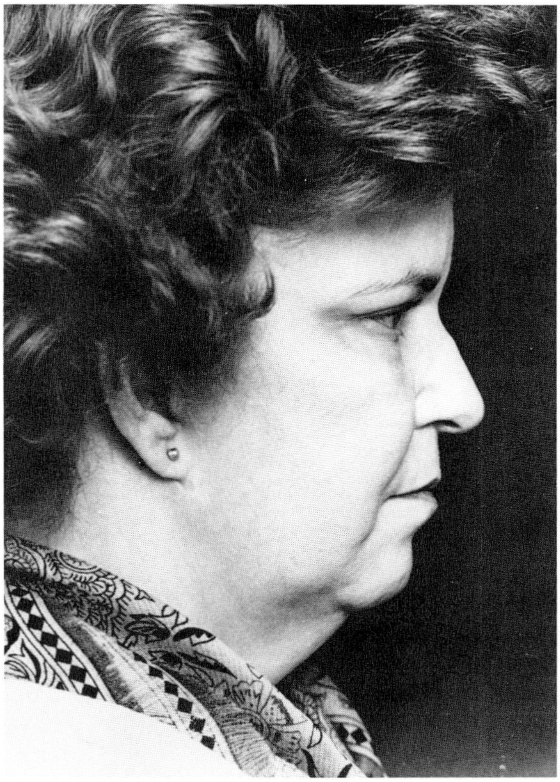
E

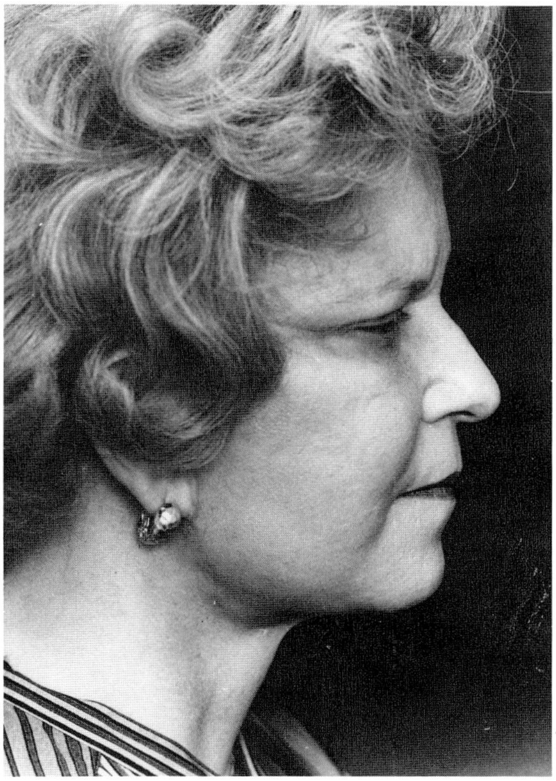
F

Figure 7–5 (continued)

midline skin and fatty fold extending from the submental crease to below the midneck crease.

INTRAOPERATIVE SEQUENCE OF THE RHYTIDECTOMY

1. Submental area (see Chapter 3):
   a. Subcutaneous fat elevated at preplatysma muscle level.
   b. Anterior borders of the platysma muscle elevated.
   c. Subplatysma muscle limited lipectomy.
   d. Resection/approximation of the anterior border of the platysma muscle.
   e. Transection/wedge removal of the platysma muscle at the cervicomental angle level (anterior border to midbody of the mandible level, approximately anterior 50%).
   f. Moderate subcutaneous fat excision on the deep surface of the skin–subcutaneous fat flap in the anterior cervical region.
2. Temporal region (see Chapter 4): Elevation of the superficial temporal fascia.
3. Cheek and posterior cervical region (see Chapter 4): Subdermal elevation of skin flaps.
4. Skin and subcutaneous fat elevation from the sternomastoid muscle to join the submental preplatysma muscle dissection (see Chapter 4).

Figure 7–5 (continued)

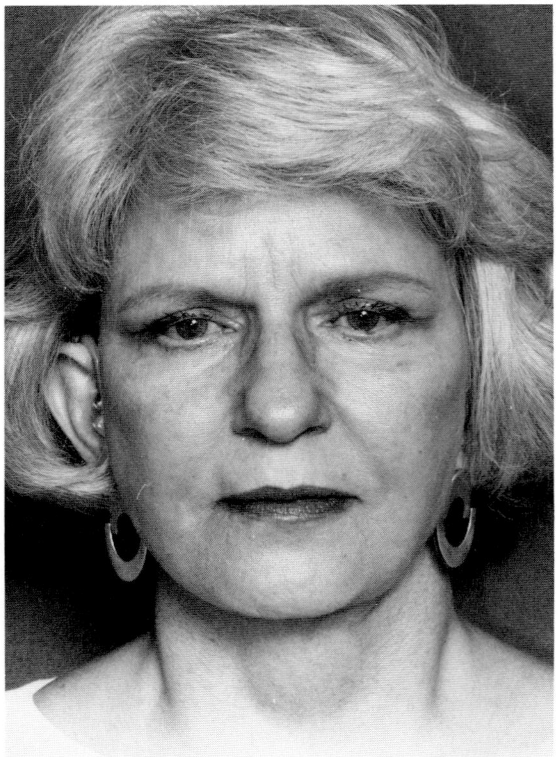

G

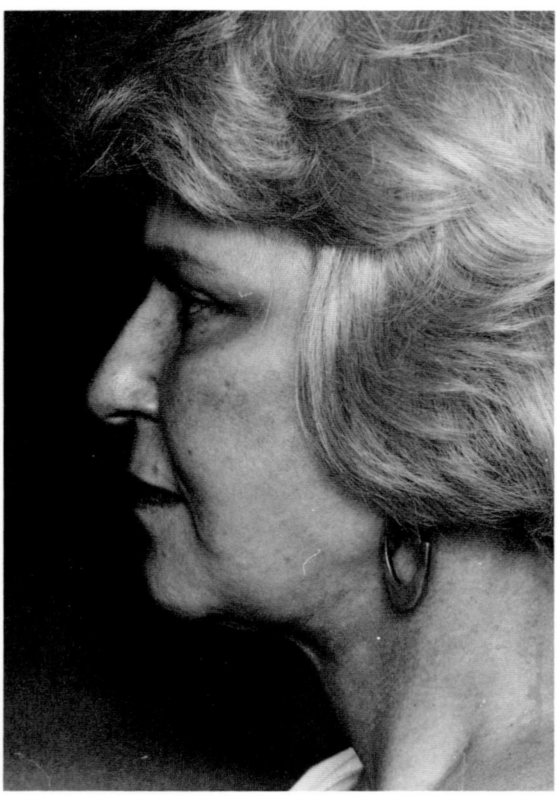

H

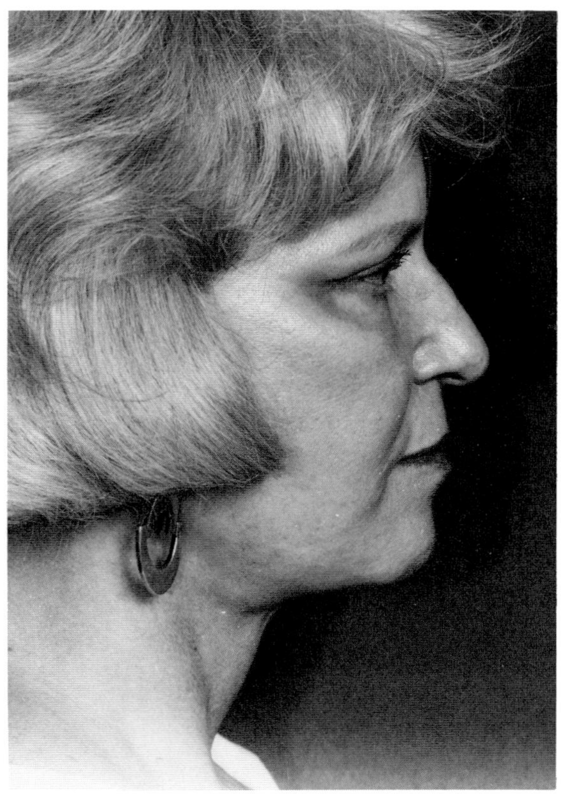

I

5. Cheek SMAS and medial subcutaneous dissection of the infraorbital area (zygomatic zone) (see Chapter 5): Extensive elevation with penetration to nasolabial fold.
6. Subtotal transection of the platysma muscle (posterior border) at the cervicomental angle level (see Chapter 5).
7. Skin redrape and closure (see Chapter 6).

Discussion

The postoperative rhytidectomy views 6 months and 6 years (Figs. 7–5B,D,F; G,H,I) show, as in Case 4, the ability to develop a cervicomental angle that maintains its contour. The lipectomy technique, pre– and postplatysma muscle, and transection of the platysma muscle from its anterior border to its midportion, or further, establish the improved appearance of the neck and mandible contour. As noted, the amount of subcutaneous fat remaining should be in equilibrium with the patient's subcutaneous fat layer elsewhere, that is, in areas where no lipectomy is performed. It is better to reoperate an area with excess fat than to have a disparity between an unoperated (no defatting) area and an overoperated (excess defatting) area that cannot be corrected. The SMAS and platysma were not reoperated on (1979–1985); however, a limited skin redrape of the face and neck was done in 1983. At that time, some fat irregularities were reduced.

The SMAS restoration even in the "heavy" face improves the nasolabial folds above the oral commissure and reduces the continuity of this fold below the commissure, which improves the mandibular line and helps eliminate the jowl.

EIGHT

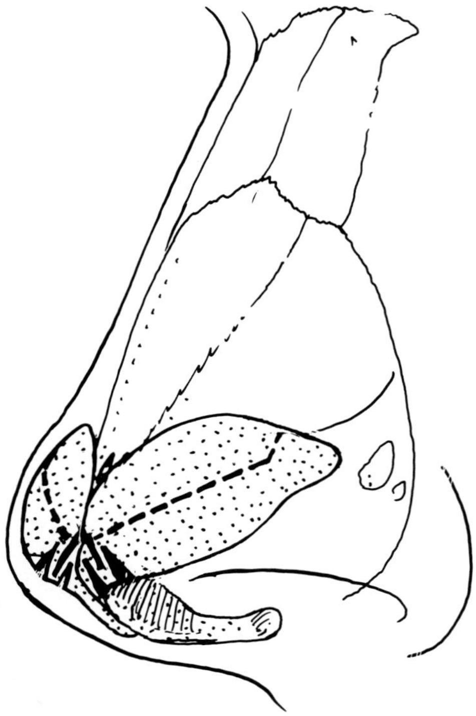

Adjunctive Procedures of the Lower Face To Enhance Rhytidectomy

A sound, reliable facelift procedure, while a vast and happy improvement for the patient, can be thought of as the foundation platform for an adjunctive procedure, which, out of proportion to its magnitude, adds a "giant leap" forward in the final overall results. In the lower face, fat contouring of the neck and jawline, augmentation of the mentum and nasal tip elevation, and/or reduction of bulbousness of the tip, when indicated, provide the ultimate restoration of the lower portion of the face to a more youthful appearance.

Many patients seeking facial restoration surgery think only in terms of a face-lift or are frightened that too much of a change will result in their "not looking like themselves." A careful and detailed explanation of the adjunctive procedure(s) advised, perhaps with some photographs, can lead to a major success, whereas without the adjunctive procedure, a superb facelift can appear to be an average result.

The cases in this chapter are presented to demonstrate the value of adjunctive procedures and no attempt is made to discuss the subject matter in detail. See Chapter 4 for a discussion of the removal of excess fat of the neck and of a technique of submental and subplatysma muscle lipectomy.

Augmentation of the Mentum

Augmentation of the mentum with a chin implant is indicated either in hypogenesis of the mentum associated with an obtuse cervicomental angle and/or excess fat in the neck, or when hypogenesis of the mentum alone exists. At times, in the absence of hypogenesis of the mentum, an obtuse cervicomental angle will be improved by minimal accentuation of the mentum.

Table 8–1 outlines the indications for augmentation mentoplasty associated with rhytidectomy. The simplest situation is mild hypogenesis of the mentum, a normal cervicomental angle, and a thin layer of subcutaneous fat.

Table 8–1. Indications for Augmentation Mentoplasty in Rhytidectomy

1. Hypogenesis of the mentum, minimal to moderate, with a satisfactory cervicomental angle
2. Hypogenesis of the mentum, minimal to moderate, associated with an obtuse cervicomental angle
3. Hypogenesis of the mentum, minimal to moderate, associated with a fatty neck
4. Hypogenesis of the mentum, minimal to moderate, associated with items 2 and 3 above

With a minimal amount of hypogenesis of the mentum, a small implant with or without wraparound extensions, depending on the shape of the mandible, improves the chin and profile contour. In this situation, a chin implant corrects the deficiency of the mentum. In the individual with a tendency of the chin to droop, or slide down from the point of the insertion on the mentum, an implant elevates the soft tissue of the mentum to a better level on the mentum, which adds to a more youthful appearance.

When there is minimal hypogenesis of the mentum in the presence of an obtuse cervicomental angle and a normal layer of the subcutaneous fat in the neck (see Table 8–1, item 2), placement of a chin implant combined with the excision of a wedge and an extended transection of the platysma muscle at the level of the cervicomental angle creates the illusion that the mandible has been lengthened and the cervicomental angle deepened. The same is true in the fatty, "heavy" neck (see Table 8–1, item 3). The subcutaneous fat is sculptured, the platysma muscle restored, and the cervicomental angle deepened by transection/resection of a horizontal wedge of the muscle at this level, and a chin implant* inserted.

The choice of the implant depends on the presenting deformity, and a trial of various implants at operation. The midline of the chin is established from the central lower or upper incisors and marked. The midline mark of the chin and the midline marker of the implant are aligned. The implant selected for the initial trial is outlined on the mentum. The mentum is approached through the submental incision by elevating the skin and subcutaneous fat from the submentum region to the inferior border of the mandible (lower border of the implant pocket). An entry port, approximately 2.5 cm in width, is established. The tissues lateral to the port along the inferior border of the mandible are left intact. Blunt and sharp dissection creates the pocket to the extent outlined on the skin. The implant is inserted and evaluated. When in the judgment of the surgeon the correction is satisfactory and the implant fits snugly in the pocket and is aligned in the midline and the horizontal plane, it is sutured in place in several locations. A 4-0 Vicryl (no. 496, Ethicon) interrupted suture is placed through the lower border of the implant and the periosteum of the mandible to secure it in the proper position. The implant pocket is closed in layers with the same suture material. This redrapes the soft tissues over the inferior border of the mandible (Fig. 8–1).

*Geniomandibular Groove Chin/Jowl Implants, McGhan Medical Corporation, Santa Barbara, CA 93111-2936

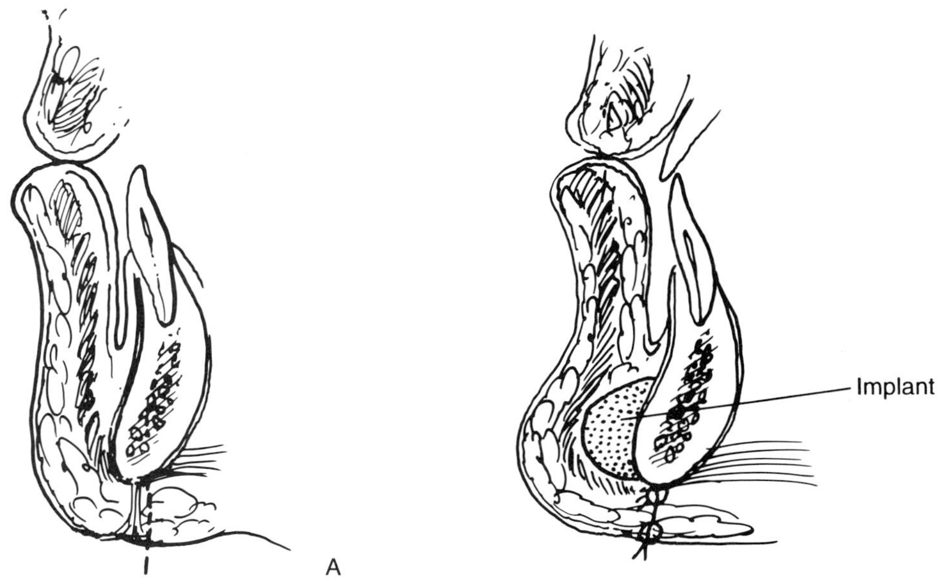

Figure 8–1. Augmentation mentoplasty for minimal hypogenesis of the mentum. **A.** Preoperative. **B.** Postoperative.

Fig. 8–2 (Case 4, see Chapter 7) illustrates a case of hypogenesis of the mentum and an obtuse cervicomental angle associated with a fatty submental skin fold of the neck (see Table 8–1, item 4). The mentum/anterior mandible was narrow. The implant selected was the medium wraparound or the extended type.* The cervicomental angle (platysma muscle) and subcutaneous fat were managed as described (see Chapter 3) and the implant inserted. The postoperative results (Fig. 8–2) show marked improvement. At the time of the preoperative consultations the patient was reluctant to accept the chin augmentation, but postoperatively was pleased she approved the suggestion.

Elevation and/or Reduction Rhinoplasty of the Nasal Tip

With aging, the lower half of the nose droops. This is a result of decreased cartilage metabolism and attenuation of the soft tissues. This detracts from a youthful appearance, whereas correction restores some of the dynamism of the facies seen in the young. If the nasal tip contours are satisfactory otherwise, simple elevation of the tip suffices to restore a diminished labial/columnella angle or a lack of tip projection. Should the tip be bulbous, or quadrilateral in shape, as well as drooped or lacking in projection, the elevation of the tip is enhanced by reducing its height and width.

A 58-year-old female (see Case 1, Chapter 7) (Fig. 8–3A, C, E) had loss of tip support and hypertrophy of the nasal tip, and attenuation of the soft tissues of the nose. The patient had no functional nasal complaints. She

*Geniomandibular Groove Chin/Jowl Implant (size 2) McGhan Medical Corporation, Santa Barbara, CA 93111-2936

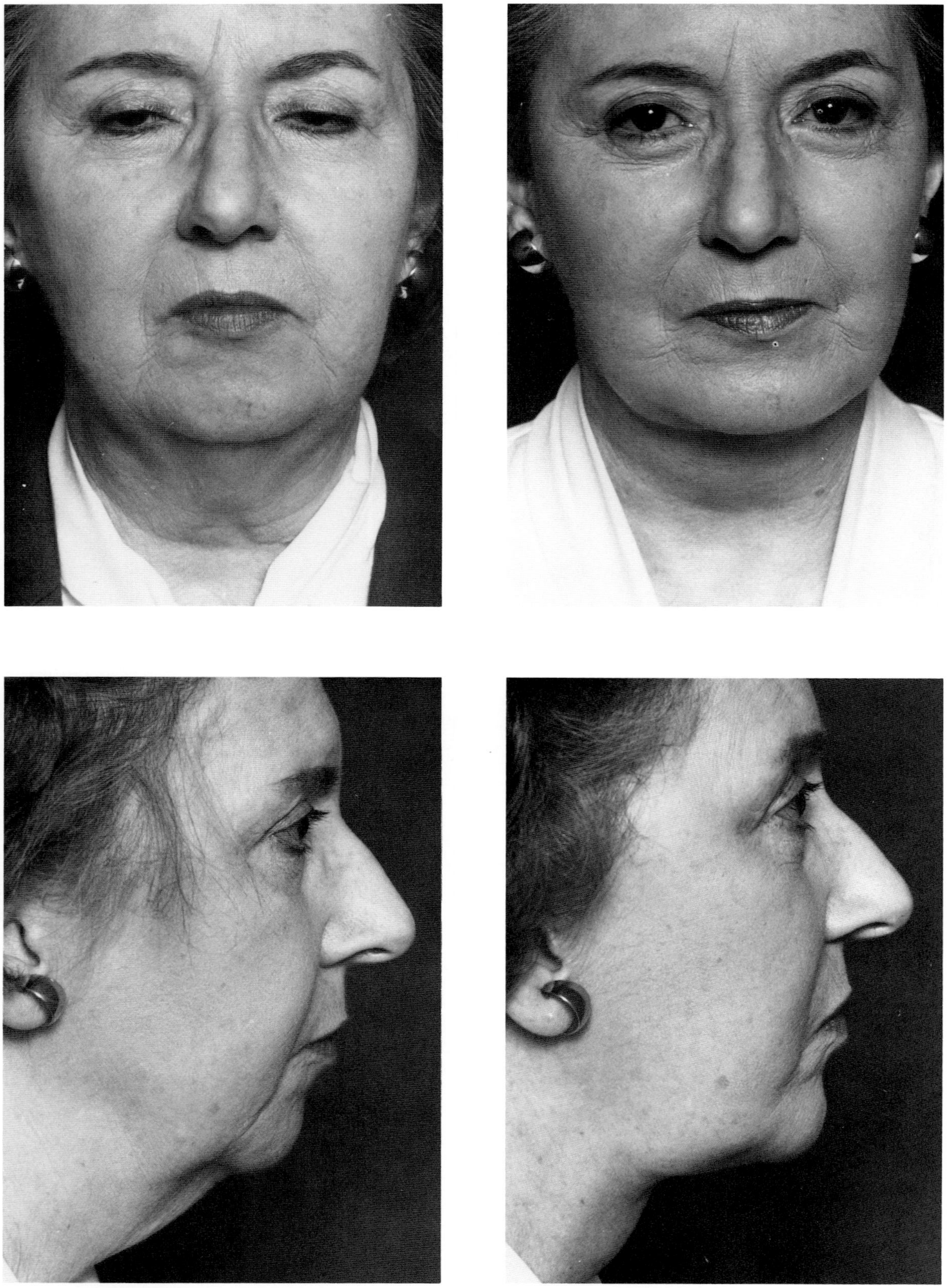

A B C D

Figure 8–2. A 62-year-old female with minimal hypogenesis of the mentum, an obtuse cervicomental angle, and a fatty fold of the neck. **A, C, E.** Before surgery. **B, D, F.** After surgery.

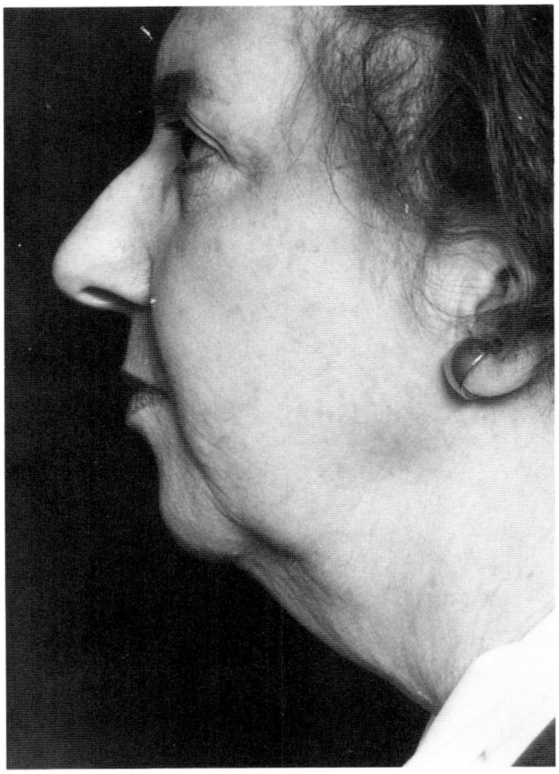
E

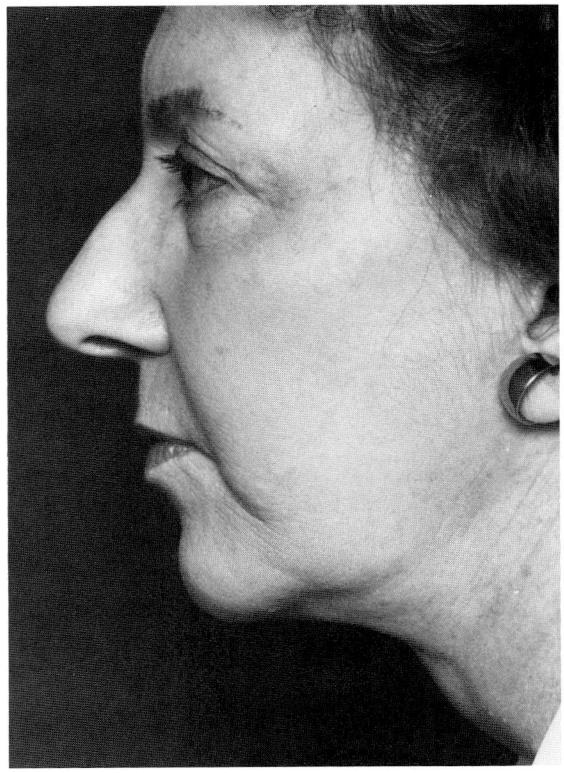
F

Figure 8–2 (continued)

accepted the suggestion that an elevation and reduction in the size of the prominent nasal tip would add to the integration of her facial surgery and achieve a more youthful and harmonious appearance.

Fig. 8–3A, C, E shows a bulbous (quadrilateral) tip with a minimal visualization of the columnella in the front view. The profile views (see Fig. 8–3C, E) show a lack of projection of the nasal tip (droop of the tip), the columnella minimally recessed, and a satisfactory columnella-labial angle (open angle). Table 8–2 outlines the surgical plan.

The lower lateral cartilages are reduced in height through infracartilaginous incisions. After reduction in the height to approximately 5 mm, the dome of the lower lateral cartilage is attenuated. Fig. 8–4A, B illustrates this, and Fig. 8–4C shows the intraoperative reduction of the lateral crus of the lower lateral nasal cartilages.

An intercartilaginous incision and transfixion incision of the membranous septum are made. The nasal skin sleeve is widely elevated. Approximately 2 mm of the caudal septum cartilage (anterior two-thirds) (Fig. 8–5A, B) and the attenuated membranous septum are reduced. The upper lateral nasal cartilages are reduced accordingly. A nasal tip cartilage graft (1.2 cm) harvested from the septum is inserted in the nasal tip (Fig. 8–6). Figure 8–3B, D, F shows the postoperative result.

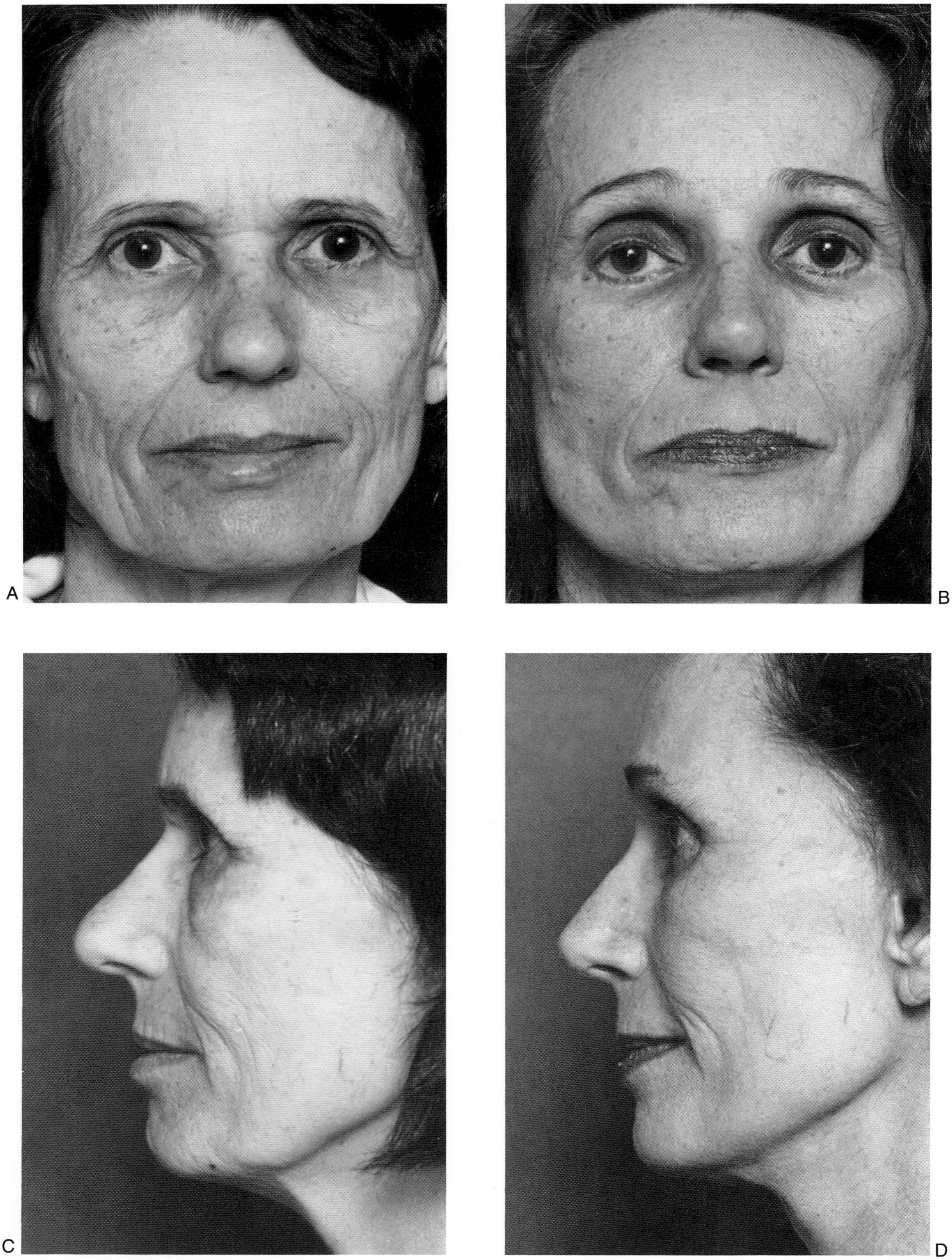

Figure 8–3. A 58-year-old female with hypertrophy of the nasal tip and lack of tip projection, preoperatively. **A, C, E.** Before surgery. **B, D, F.** After surgery.

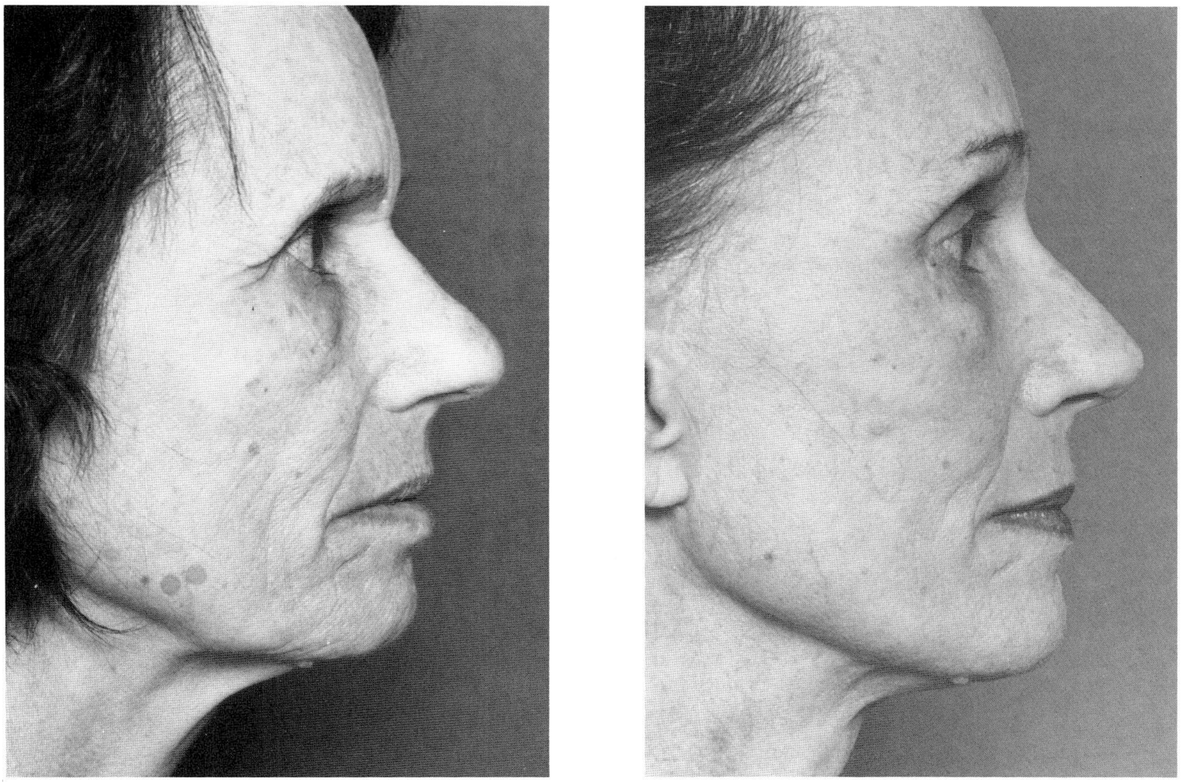

E F

Figure 8–3 (continued)

Table 8–2. The Surgical Plan

1. Reduction of height and attenuation of the dome of the lower lateral cartilages of the nose through infracartilaginous incisions
2. Intercartilaginous incisions with transfixion incision of the membranous septum
3. Wide elevation of the nasal skin sleeve
4. Excision of the attenuated membranous septum
5. Excision of 2 mm of the caudal septum, anterior two-thirds, including the vestibule skin
6. Submucous resection of 2 mm of the lower border of the upper lateral nasal cartilages
7. Harvest of septal cartilage
8. Insertion of a septal cartilage nasal tip graft

Figure 8–4. The reduction of the height and attenuation of the dome of the lower lateral nasal cartilage. **A.** Illustration of the reduction of the lower lateral nasal cartilages and attenuation of the dome of the medial and lateral crura. **B.** Illustration of photograph (C).

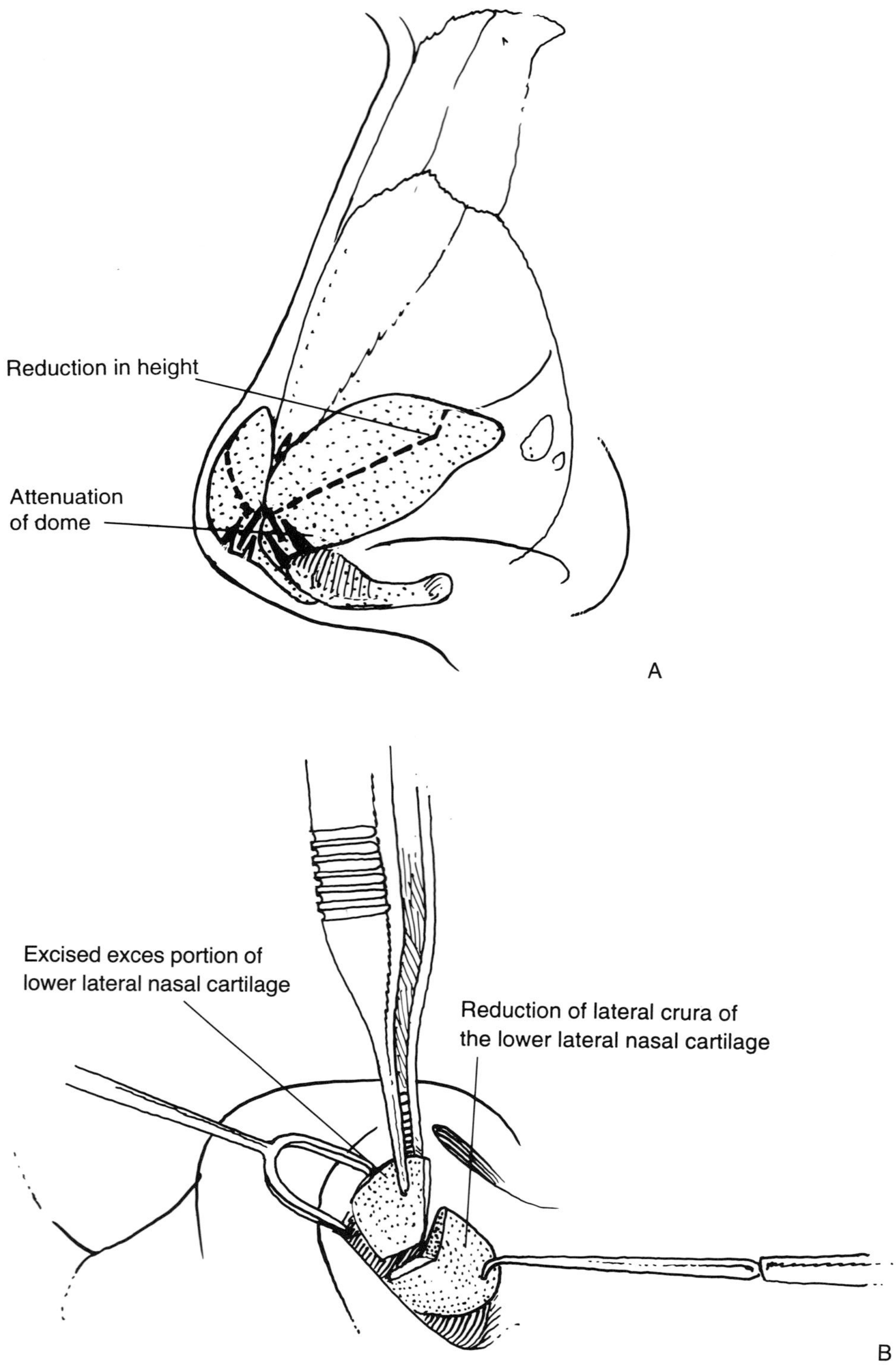

Figure 8–4 (continued) **C.** Intraoperative.

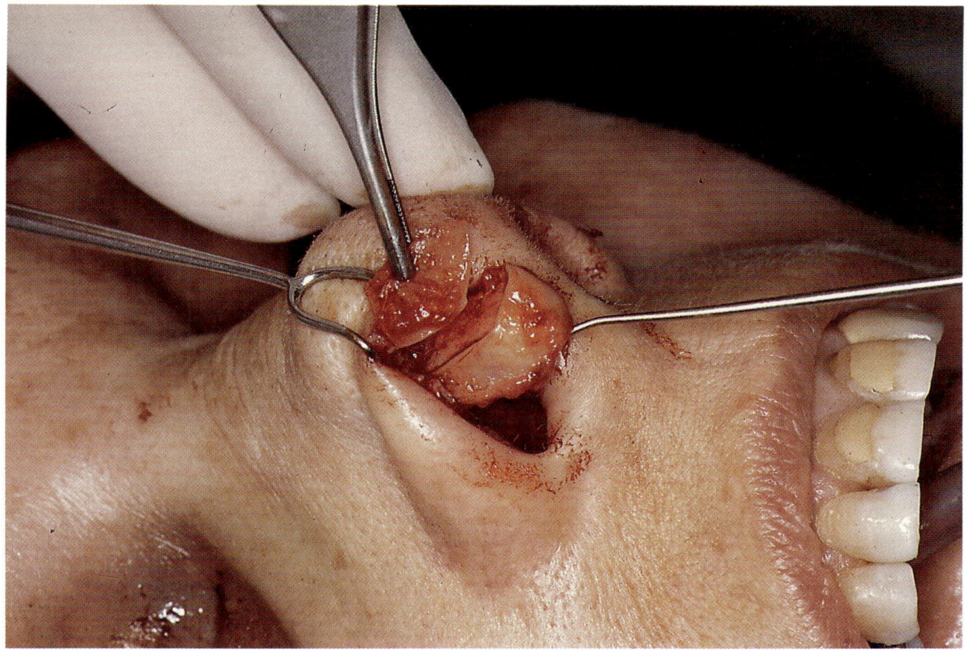
C

Figure 8–5. Excision of 2 mm of the anterior two-thirds of the caudal septum and the attenuated membranous septum. **A.** Illustration of photograph (B).

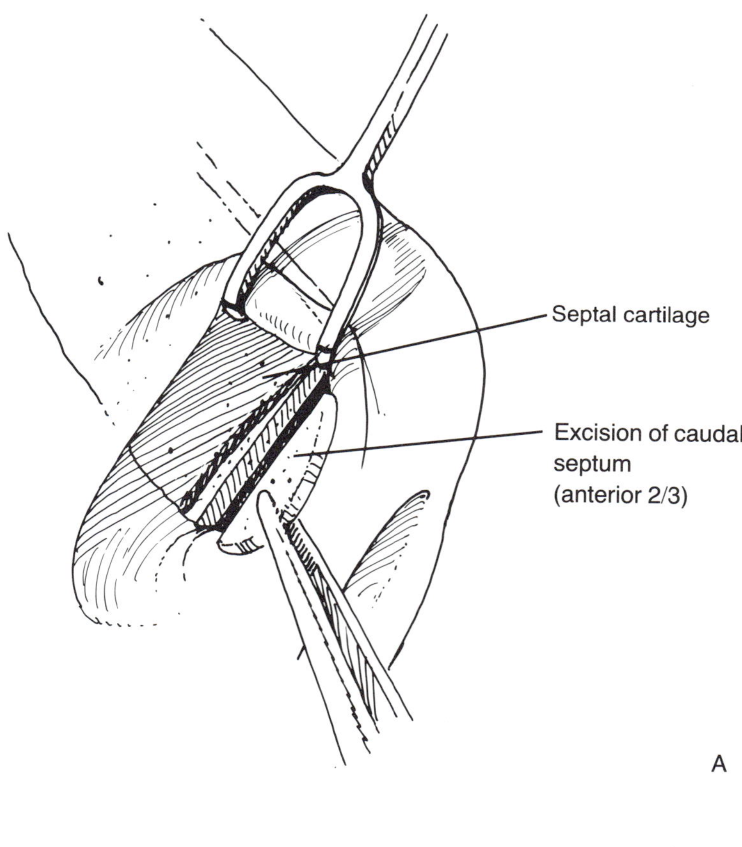

A

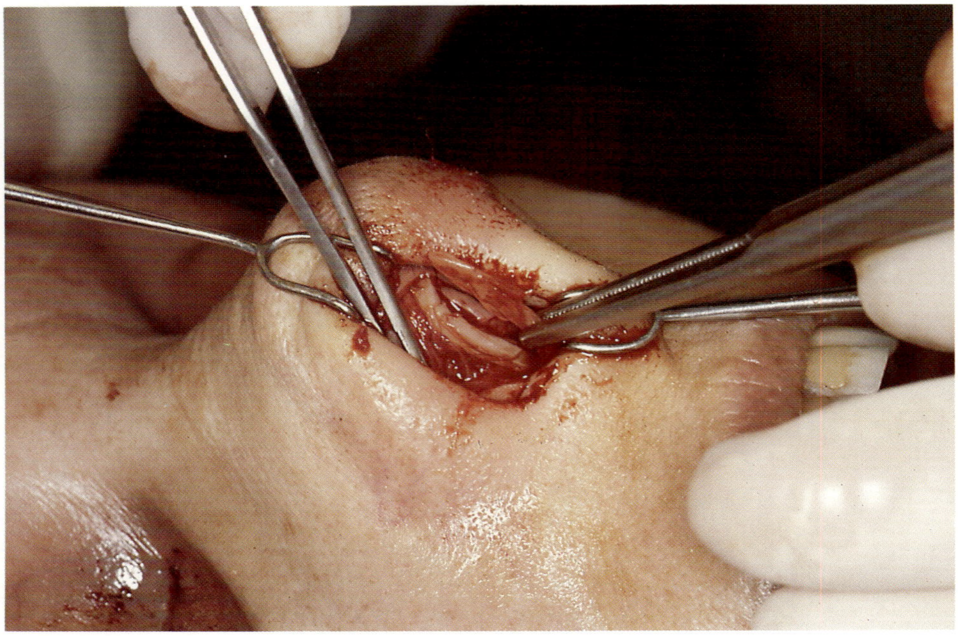

B

Figure 8–5 (continued) **B.** Intraoperative.

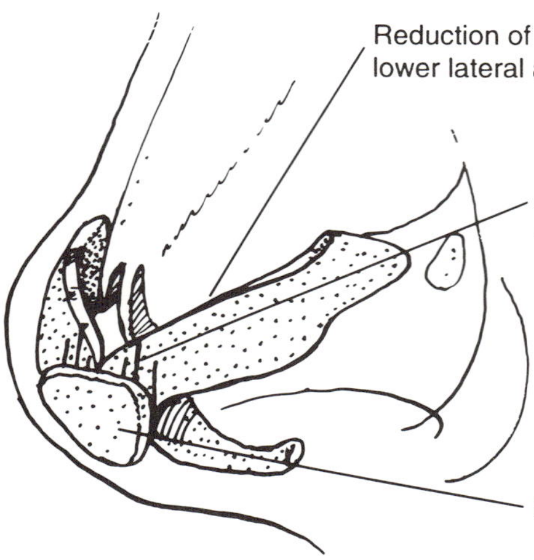

A

Figure 8–6. The nasal tip graft. **A.** Illustration of nasal tip graft.

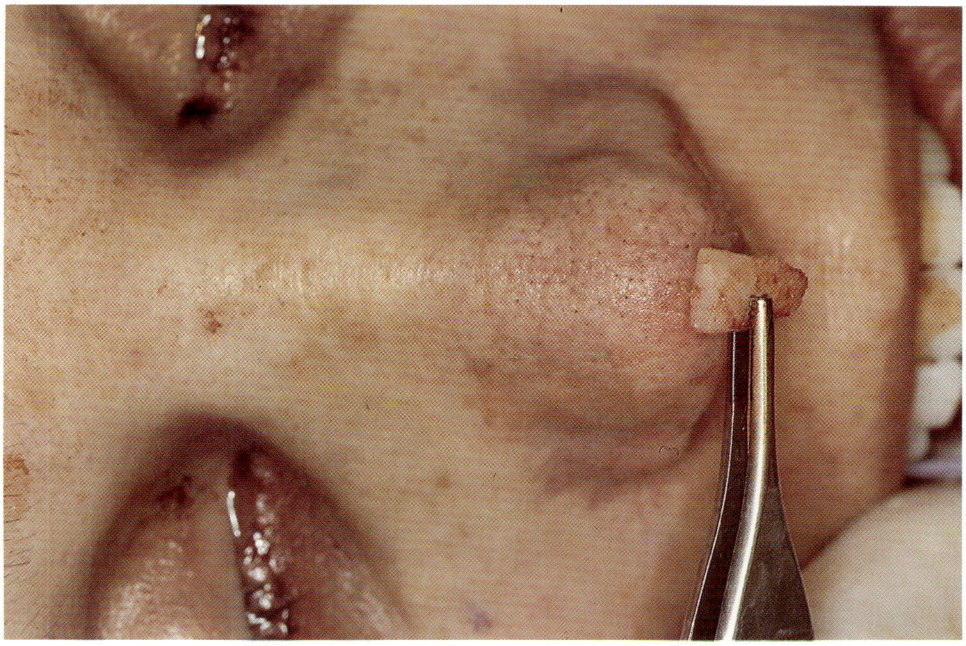

B

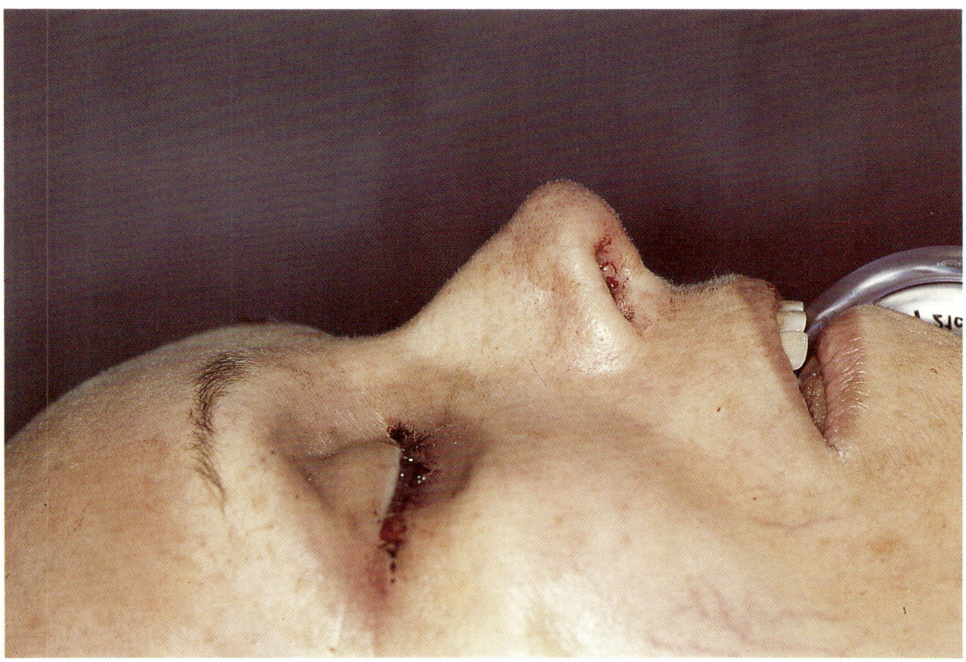

C

Figure 8–6 (continued) **B.** Nasal tip graft, 1.2 cm, prepared for insertion. **C.** Nasal tip graft in place.

INDEX